WITHDRAWN

EPIDEMICS
in the
MODERN
WORLD

Twayne's

LITERATURE
&
SOCIETY
SERIES

Leo Marx, General Editor
Massachusetts Institute of Technology

810.9
K893e

EPIDEMICS
in the
MODERN
WORLD

Joann P. Krieg

Twayne Publishers • New York
MAXWELL MACMILLAN CANADA • TORONTO
MAXWELL MACMILLAN INTERNATIONAL • NEW YORK OXFORD SINGAPORE SYDNEY

Twayne's Literature & Society Series No. 3

Epidemics in the Modern World

Joann P. Krieg

Copyright © 1992 by Twayne Publishers

All rights reserved. No part of this book may be reproduced or transmitted in any form or by any means, electronic or mechanical, including photocopying, recording, or by any information storage and retrieval system, without permission in writing from the Publisher.

Twayne Publishers
Macmillan Publishing Company
866 Third Avenue
New York, New York 10022

Maxwell Macmillan Canada, Inc.
1200 Eglinton Avenue East
Suite 200
Don Mills, Ontario M3C 3N1

Macmillan Publishing Company is part of the Maxwell Communication Group of Companies.

Library of Congress Cataloging-in-Publication Data

Krieg, Joann P.
Epidemics in the modern world / Joann P. Krieg.
p.   cm.—(Twayne's literature & society series ; no. 3)
Includes bibliographical references and index.
ISBN 0-8057-8852-2 (hc : alk. paper)—ISBN
0-8057-8859-X (pb : alk. paper)
1. Epidemiology—United States.   2. Social medicine.
3. Literature and medicine.   I. Title.   II. Series.
RA650.5.K75   1992
614.4'973—dc20   92-14090
CIP

The paper used in this publication meets the minimum requirements of American National Standard for Information Sciences—Permanence of Paper for Printed Library Materials. ANSI Z3948-1984.⊚™

10 9 8 7 6 5 4 3 2 1 (hc)

10 9 8 7 6 5 4 3 2 1 (pb)

Printed in the United States of America

For John

CAT Oct 4 '93

7-20-83 FBS 25.33

ALLEGHENY COLLEGE LIBRARY

CONTENTS

FOREWORD

Each volume in the Literature and Society Series examines the interplay between a body of writing and an historical event. By "event" we mean a circumscribable episode, located in a specific time and place; it may be an election, a royal reign, a presidency, a war, a revolution, a voyage of discovery, a trial, an engineering project, a scientific innovation, a social movement, an invention, a law, or an epidemic. But it must have given rise to a substantial corpus of interpretive writing.

The idea of elucidating the relations between writing and its historical context is not new. In the past, however, those relations too often have been treated as merely ancillary, static, or unidirectional. Historians have drawn on literary works chiefly in order to illustrate, corroborate, or enliven an essentially socioeconomic or political narrative; or, by the same token, literary scholars have introduced a summary of extraliterary events chiefly in order to provide an historical setting—a kind of theatrical "backdrop"—for their discussions of a body of writing.

In this series, however, the aim is to demonstrate how knowledge of events and an understanding of what has been written about them enhance each other. Each is more meaningful in the presence of, than apart from, the other. Just as history can only be created by acts of interpretation, so any written work invariably bears the marks of the historical circumstances in which it was composed. The controlling principle of the Literature and Society Series is the reciprocal relation between our conception of events and the writing they may be said to have provoked.

Leo Marx

PREFACE

The story of the American experience cannot always be told in the positive, upbeat tone we most like to hear. There are those aspects of human life that, even in a democracy, exercise a kind of tyranny over the lives and fortunes of innocent victims. Of the four legendary horsemen who are said to periodically establish their empire over human history—War, Famine, Pestilence, and Death—Pestilence is probably the most feared for its repugnant horrors. With good cause has this evil long been associated in humankind's collective consciousness with retribution, divine or otherwise, for falling short of the mark by which we are judged.

For centuries stories and histories bore witness to the plagues of Europe and of regions beyond, plagues that, it was hoped, would be eluded when the New World beckoned. The very remoteness of the New World's geography, set off from other land masses as it was, like Sir Thomas More's Utopia, seemed to guarantee its immunity to the winds of pestilence that might blow elsewhere. Yet even here they blew, whispering, in the words of Death, that other horseman of the apocalypse, "*Et in Arcadia, ego*" ("And here too, in the ideal world, I am present"). This is the story of some of the epidemics that have swept, and still do sweep, that portion of the New World known as the United States of America.

My interest in this topic began with Charles Brockden Brown's fictional depictions of the yellow fever epidemics of the 1790s. The more I researched that episode in the nation's history and Brown's involvement in it, the more

I realized the similarity between much of what happened then in the United States and what Michel Foucault describes in *The Birth of the Clinic* (1973). The same potential existed late in the eighteenth century in the United States, as in France, for the development of an abusive power. And it would have been just as easily gained from the observational method in medicine that Foucault delineates, since epidemics threaten social order and invite control mechanisms wherever they occur. The potential was even greater in the case of the yellow fever epidemics because of the threat they presented to the continuance of the nation, then in the first decade of its existence. Heavily dependent on immigration for its work force and on trade for its economy, the country was in no position to close its ports in the face of epidemic; nor could it afford to pronounce itself the source of infection. Much depended upon the rationalist influence of the medical profession and its observations of the epidemical fever.

In his subsequent study, *Discipline and Punish: The Birth of the Prison* (1977), Foucault traces the broadening of the scientific control mechanism gained in France as a result of empirical medicine; the physician's gaze evolved into the surveillance techniques of penal institutions. As I expanded my own investigation into the yellow fever epidemics and other episodes of epidemical disease in the United States, however, I found an essential difference between what occurred here and the French experience. Because of his concentration on France, Foucault's theorizing excludes the democratic experience of rational observation, what might be called the collective eye of social control. His conclusions are drawn from the workings of an autocratic society and need the perspective of his nineteenth-century *compatriote*, Alexis de Tocqueville, to throw light on the workings of democracy. In his classic work *Democracy in America* (1835), Tocqueville expressed concern that the cause of freedom might be undermined in a democracy by what he labeled "the tyranny of the majority." Clearly such a tyranny could have developed and might well have taken on those aspects of power Foucault uncovers in the France of Tocqueville's time. (Indeed, Tocqueville visited the United States to gain information on the penitentiary system inaugurated here; much of what Foucault describes, then, stems from prison theories as current in America as in Europe.) But the young French aristocrat also recognized in the American impulse toward what he termed "associationism," or collective action, the possibility for a minority to counter the power of the majority and exert an influence on the mechanism of social control.

With this difference in mind, then, the questions that governed my investigation became, How does the majority respond to epidemics in America? and, What happens to minorities at such a critical time? Since my interest is in both the history of the epidemics and their representation in literature, a further question arose: What does literature contribute to the record? In chapter 1 I offer a schematic of the answers my investigation yielded, and in succeeding chapters, the evidence for these answers drawn from the record of specific epidemics furnished by history and literature.

When my interest in epidemics was awakened by reading Brown's romances of the early Republic, the idea of a nation, especially the United States of America, being threatened by epidemic seemed remote. If ever there were a nation that typifies the modern world it is the USA, and epidemical diseases are always dealt with in the modern world by developing a vaccine. Or so I thought. But the modern world has been brought up short by a virus that it cannot understand sufficiently to develop a preventative vaccine, and the United States is one of two epicenters of occurrence for that virus—HIV, the virus that produces AIDS. May that understanding come quickly.

I am grateful to Princeton University Libraries for permission to quote Philip Freneau's "Pestilence," in *The Poems of Philip Freneau*, vol. 3, edited by Fred Lewis Pattee (Princeton University Library, 1907). For their part in helping me with this work I wish to thank Edward Chalfant, Lisa MacLeman, Gene Stith, Gary La Rosa, John Mauro, and Barbara Dastoor. The Center for Scholarly Research at Hofstra University provided time for its preparation.

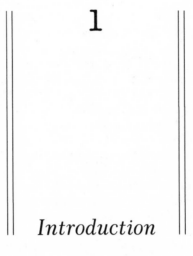

1

Introduction

THERE ARE FEW WORDS THAT HAVE THE POWER TO CONJURE images as vivid as those aroused by the word *epidemic*. For centuries the word, along with others of equally compelling force such as *plague* and *pestilence*, registered on the mind as a powerful indicator of human impotence in the face of what appeared to be divine will. Attempts to fathom the mystery of these apparently divinely ordained occurrences led to all manner of speculation as to the immediate causes of certain epidemics in given places at specific times. Thus, in the fourteenth century Jews, heretics, and witches were blamed for the plague that swept Europe and were put to death in the hope that doing so would purge the remaining faithful of the corrupting influences that brought death to the body and the soul.

World literature offers many works, including not a few masterworks, that present stirring narratives and often horrifying images of peoples trapped by epidemics. Giovanni Boccaccio's *The Decameron* (1349–51) is a collection of stories told as amusement to while away time spent in exile from Florence while the plague ravaged that Italian city in the fourteenth century. Daniel

Defoe's *Journal of the Plague Year* (1722) is an eighteenth-century retrospective account of London during the plague of 1665. Tuberculosis, of epidemic proportions in nineteenth-century Europe and America, has left us not only images—of Alexandre Dumas's *La Dame aux camélias* (1852) and Thomas Mann's sanitorium patients in *The Magic Mountain* (1924)—by which to remember that outbreak but also sounds—Mimi's racking cough in Giacomo Puccini's *La Bohème* (1896) and Violetta's last, exultant cry of rebirth before succumbing to the disease in Giuseppe Verdi's *La Traviata* (1853). In *Death in Venice* (1912) Mann depicts the effect of epidemical disease on the individual, and in *The Plague* (1948), Albert Camus shows its effect on a community.

Absent from such a list of literary works dealing with epidemics is any contribution by an American writer. One could offer numerous reasons for this, including the most obvious one—that American literature has tended to reflect the nation's struggle to become its own subject. One might even be tempted to claim that epidemical disease has not been part of the nation's history, and that American writers have not chosen to treat the subject of epidemics in other countries. But the first assertion would not be true, though the inference might be drawn from the very paucity it seeks to explain. America *has* been visited by epidemics, often and repeatedly—as in the three separate cholera visitations of the nineteenth century—but as this study reveals, the nation's authors have chosen for the most part either to ignore these occurrences or, in writing of them, to disguise their subject. The reasons for the denial and the obfuscation have to do with national pride and economic fear, motives that have impelled humans almost as long as epidemics have plagued them and that are tied in with the advance of science in the modern world. The object of this study is first, to examine the historical record of epidemics in America, and second, to discover the interplay between the historical events and their literary interpretations. In most cases this involves a considerable exploration of the literary texts and the contexts in which they were produced, contexts that extend sometimes into the lives of the authors, sometimes into the life of the nation. The exploration is necessitated by the reluctance of American writers to confront directly the issues of contagion and epidemic disease, a reluctance that hinges, in many instances, on the almost mythical conception of America as having its origin outside the boundaries of human and natural history.

= A New World of Nature =

Modern history presents a very different picture of disease from that offered by the fourteenth century: it provides a record of almost unfailing success in dealing with those diseases that, in earlier times, swept through whole populations. The record begins in the first half of the eighteenth century with the introduction into European medicine of the practice of smallpox inoculation, borrowed from the traditional folk medicine of Africa and Asia. Indeed, the scientific advance gained with the introduction of smallpox inoculation was a turning point in human history, for it placed disease, even the most terrifyingly lethal and infectious diseases, within the realm of those conditions susceptible to human remedy. With such power at their command, whole masses of people could begin to view their world in the same way as did the more learned among them, those rationalist philosophers and adherents of Lockean empiricism who posited a worldly environment amenable to modification by human design.

It is this view that for the purposes of this study defines the modern world. Our story of epidemics in America begins in colonial Boston with the struggle, described in chapter 2, between an unlikely supporter of inoculation, the quintessential Puritan Cotton Mather, and the *New-England Courant*, a Boston newspaper owned and printed by the Franklin brothers, James and Benjamin. Chapter 2 also examines a tale written by Nathaniel Hawthorne 100 years later for which Boston's 1721 epidemic is the setting. In his usual manner of suggesting rather than stating his theme outright, Hawthorne alludes to the epidemic as a precursor of revolution, all the while maintaining an ambiguous stance as to the source of infection. Despite its shadowy ambiguity and indirection, the tale effectively links the achievements of science to the expansion of the political imagination that produced a world picture from which both the ancient scourges of smallpox and tyranny could be banished.

In such a world there seemed little that humans could not come to know and understand through the application of their own reason. A young Jeremy Bentham, thrilled by advances in knowledge of the natural world, hailed his age, in 1776, as one that "teems with discovery and with improvement."[1] Not only could they know and shape the world in which they lived, but humans themselves could be changed, made more perfect. And so, in the same year that Bentham voiced in England his jubilation at the advance of knowledge, Thomas Jefferson drafted the Declaration of Independence, which advanced the notion that humans might govern themselves. It was in this climate of thought that the dream of American democracy was realized, and a future unclouded by the evils that for centuries had attended human existence seemed to beckon.

But the realization of the dream was not totally unattended by reminders of a past that included, among other evils, diseases capable of wiping out thousands within a few weeks or months. As if a reminder of human limitations, yellow fever struck the eastern seacoast cities of the new Republic almost every year in the final decade of the eighteenth century. Despite its regular appearances, the disease remained a mystery. Arriving so soon after the creation of the United States of America that it threatened to expunge the fledgling democracy, yellow fever dominated for a time the lives of Americans living in the most populated region of the country. Doctors in the affected cities bent all their efforts toward discovering the cause of the disease and the most effective treatment, but to no avail. In frustration they fell to fighting among themselves over competing theories, and in the highly volatile political atmosphere of the time their medical factions quickly broadened to embrace the growing national partisanship that soon after gave rise to the party system in government.

In time the annual epidemics subsided (without the doctors ever having learned their cause), but they left Americans with strong doubts about the safety of their natural environment, doubts that, for the sake of national unity and pride, had to be repressed. This need also created an atmosphere in which American writers were required either to ignore those aspects of American life that indicated a less than ideal environment, or to refer to them obliquely by resorting to analogous situations or topics.

It is difficult to fault early Americans for wishing to avoid acknowledging their country as the source of epidemic fevers unknown in Europe. No one likes to think about epidemic disease, and no country wishes to be labeled its source, least of all a country that imagined itself immune to many of Europe's evils by reason of isolation and a divine providence. Indeed, much of the myth of American innocence promulgated in the nineteenth century was informed by this twin claim to immunity despite the fact that the claim did not readily accommodate the historical record of infection, contagion, and epidemic disease within the nation's borders. It may be that the myth of innocence is examined repeatedly in American literature, from the early romanticism of Charles Brockden Brown to the realism of Henry James, partly because of this contradiction.

Simplistic reasoning would see in the reluctance of Americans to deal straightforwardly with their history of epidemical diseases little more than the kind of nationalism that often led European nations to identify such diseases with countries other than their own as a way of attaching blame and of dissociating themselves. Thus syphilis was "the French disease" in Spain, and "the Spanish disease" in France. But America's reaction to epidemics is made up of more complex psychological elements, a result of the nation's peculiar sense of itself as the site of the second Paradise, or, in Puritan theology, the New Jerusalem. The denial of epidemic disease originating within its borders surely stems from the American fear that the presence of such evils would cast doubt on the New World as the probable locus for these sacred precincts. A hundred years after the 1721 smallpox epidemic Hawthorne was still sufficiently under the influence of his Puritan background to feel conflicted about the degree to which revolution might be considered a concomitant of the kind of breakdown of social order that accompanies epidemics. That he cloaks his conflict in a veil of romance is the sign of an insistence, originating with the earlier writer, Charles Brockden Brown, that truth lies not in the realm of pure reason but in the regions of romance, with its acceptance of the darker aspects of life. Those darker aspects include the capacity for self-deception and error, two dimensions of the human experience that the rationalists did not always concede; but they also pointed to the romantic conceptions of light *and* dark, good *and* evil, upon which rested the idea of America as the disputed landscape where goodness and virtue would triumph.

Charles Brockden Brown's personal experience of the yellow fever epidemics in the 1790s has provided American literature with its earliest, and most historically accurate, depiction of pestilence abroad in the land. *Arthur Mervyn, or, Memoirs of the Year 1793* (1799–1800) includes scenes of Philadelphia, then the nation's capital, to rival Defoe's plague-ridden London. A reading of his *Edgar Huntly* (1799), offered in chapter 3 of this study, discovers there a yellow fever subtext that opposes the argument presented in *Arthur Mervyn*. The disagreement of texts arises from the conflict between reason and romance as ways of knowing truth: *Edgar Huntly* is as grounded in the author's need to preserve the sense of mystery and romance in human experience as *Arthur Mervyn* is in his need to rationally dispel the association of America with a new form of plague.

In the minds of Americans, epidemics—and even some forms of simple diseases, such as scurvy—were firmly associated with the Old World and its social ills and were viewed as part of the general economic deprivation and political oppression that emigrants left behind when they fled Europe for America. Propaganda used to encourage colonization from the time of the first explorers, and their "true relations" of what they had seen in the New World, emphasized purity of air and water along with natural plenty. Later, the eighteenth-century immigrant J. Hector St. John de Crèvecoeur answered his question "What Is an American?"—an essay in *Letters from an American Farmer* (1782)—by pointing to the wholesomeness of lives rooted in economic abundance. The agricultural basis of this definition placed the American in a relationship heavily dependent upon nature in a portion of the world looked upon by European natural historians as "disgraced." The theological implication of that word was not unintended, for it was the contention of the foremost among these naturalists—Georges Louis Leclerc, Comte de Buffon—that the New World had been created after the rest of the world, by which time the life-giving molecules of nature had lost most of their energy so that nothing in the New World reached its full growth potential. Buffon further claimed that the absence of human life from much of the New World for so long a time had allowed the accumulation of fetid air and noxious vapors, which were the causes of deadly diseases.

Buffon's *Histoire naturelle* (1749–1804) (all 44 volumes!) sold widely in the United States and in France, but Americans were keenly aware of the power of such views to fashion conventionally accepted truth, and they attempted to counter them in whatever way possible. Jefferson's *Notes on the State of Virginia* (1785), written between the years 1781 and 1784, was among the first of many descriptions of American landscape designed to contradict the prevailing European view. The felt need to offset European claims that all species in the New World were stunted by nature's inability to bring them to fruition resulted in a habit of exaggeration among Americans and the invention of a folklore that emphasized the bigness of everything—landscape, animals, and humans. In the nineteenth century the justly famous Hudson River school of American landscape painting, which presented to the eye vast panoramic views of nature, was as much a political as an artistic statement and taught Americans to affirm that which they had in abundance—nature. From art to philosophy was not too great a leap, and Americans soon were being told by Ralph Waldo Emerson to look not only to nature but at it for self-knowledge, and he described for them his own emotions when in nature of being "a transparent eyeball . . . part and parcel of God."[2] There has seldom been a time and place so devoted to the theory of optics, or one that so privileged the faculty of sight, as nineteenth-century America. Whatever other influences may have been at work to produce this effect, such as scientific achievement, surely one of the most powerful was the negative view of the New World environment as it registered on the eyes of European naturalists.

Regrettably, one of the observable phenomena that lent credence to the nonsense being offered by Buffon and others was the presence in the New World of epidemical fevers unknown in Europe. Such fevers had frequently swept the colonies, but they had not created the same havoc as smallpox, and so it was the latter disease that earlier claimed the greater attention. After inoculation provided a defense against smallpox, this attention was turned to the various unclassified fevers that struck in America, often with a high degree of predictability. Michel Foucault, the French structuralist who has illuminated the connections between medical practices in eighteenth-century France and many of the subsequent attempts at social reform undertaken in that country and others, including the United States, has pointed out that, at the time, "the fundamental act of medical knowledge was the drawing up of a 'map': a symptom was situated within a disease, a disease in a specific *ensemble*, and this *ensemble* in a general plan of the pathological world."[3] Similarly (though Foucault does not address American history), it can be seen that in the early years of the new American Republic Europe's natural historians drew a map of the New World in which the symptom, fever of unknown origin, was situated within the general ensemble of a rebellious people in a disgraced landscape. In chapter 3 I discuss the introduction of the medical "spot map" in America at the time of the yellow fever epidemics as both the result of such theoretical cartography and an attempt to alter its findings.

The mapping of disease was but one aspect of an empiricism based largely on the act of seeing that came to dominate medicine in eighteenth-century France. In *Birth of the Clinic* Foucault has described the system of clinical observation by which the body of the diseased came under *le regard*, or the physician's gaze. This clinical approach to disease was part of a generalized epistemological shift that began in the seventeenth century and ushered in the age of modern medicine. No longer was knowledge located in abstract universals but in directly observable natural phenomena. In medicine disease became located within the body of the patient rather than within a system of disease categories.

The inherent danger of the physician's gaze is its potential for the kind of intrusive surveillance that Foucault has delineated, but the enormous good derived from direct medical observation as advocated by the Parisian school of clinical treatment must not pass unnoted. In America its influence was felt in ways that have not been fully appreciated or understood, though the story of one American doctor trained in this method—who was also a writer— is part of the history of epidemics in this country. Overshadowed by the later pronouncement of the obstetrician Ignaz Semmelweis in Austria, the work of Dr. Oliver Wendell Holmes in the field of puerperal fever remains a major American contribution to medical science generally, and to the understanding of contagion specifically.

= Dr. Holmes and Puerperal Fever =

In 1843, four years before Ignaz Semmelweis incurred the wrath of the Viennese medical establishment by publicly proclaiming that doctors were themselves carriers of the deadly puerperal, or childbed fever, Oliver Wendell Holmes read a paper before the Boston Society for Medical Improvement in which he made the identical accusation. Holmes had no knowledge of Dr. Semmelweis's work, nor did he claim originality for the idea: he cited others who earlier had noted the high death rate of women delivered by certain midwives. Holmes made the logical leap of understanding that these midwives were carrying the sepsis of childbed fever from sick mothers to well mothers, acting as vectors. Doctors did the same thing, Holmes insisted; moreover, they could initiate the fever by attending a woman in labor after tending someone with a serious infection or after performing an autopsy on an infected body.

American obstetricians received this insight with the same ill grace shown by their Viennese counterparts toward Semmelweis a few years later. (Semmelweis was hounded out of the medical profession and died in a mental hospital.) American obstetricians had more ammunition, however: the target of their ridicule was but 34 years old and a dabbler in poetry. But Holmes came of a good Boston family that had the means to educate him—after he abandoned his original course of study in law—at a private medical school in Boston and at Harvard. He did well at these institutions but was unwilling to accept licensing at the end of the course work. Holmes was intelligent enough to recognize the provincialism of American medicine and to know where to look for something more. He persuaded his father to finance further study in Paris, and in 1833 he began a two-year course that took him out of the classroom and brought him directly into contact with the sick.

The clinical practices of the French doctors were what Holmes considered truly "scientific," unlike the practices of American doctors who (in the style of the previous century's Benjamin Rush) bled and purged their patients in the belief that some action was better than none even if, as often happened, the patient was too weak to survive the treatment. At the end of the two years Holmes returned to Boston, took his medical degree from Harvard, and entered practice; but his medical outlook had been set by his Paris experience, and he was never at ease with his fellow physicians. It was in large part resentment of his difference from them that caused the furor over his puerperal fever paper, but it was also his suggested rules for preventing the transmission of the fever via their own persons. Doctors were not accustomed to having their peers establish rules and regulations for them to follow, and Holmes deeply affronted them with his concluding point: "Whatever indulgence may be granted to those who have heretofore been the ignorant causes of so much misery, the time has come when the existence of a *private pestilence* in the sphere of a single physician should be looked upon, not as a misfortune, but a crime; and in the knowledge of such occurrences the duties of the practitioner to his profession should give way to his paramount obligations to society."[4]

The idea of being considered "a private pestilence" (the phrase has been borrowed for the title of chapter 6 in the present work) was more than a little unsettling to the members of the Boston medical community, and they reacted with a violence that would have shaken a man less grounded in the principles of science than was this product of the Paris clinics. Holmes's response to their vituperation was characteristic of him and may have provided the germ of an idea that later found its way into the writing of another New Englander, Henry David Thoreau. When Holmes was under attack he maintained his position by declaring: "When facts are numerous, and unquestionable, and unequivocal in their significance, theory must follow them as best it may, keeping time with their step; and not go before them, marching to the sound of its own drum and trumpet."[5]

Of his Paris studies Holmes has much to say in his journals, mostly about the eccentricities of his teachers; later, in a reminiscence, he remarks that too much of his time in Paris "was lost in ill-directed study." He claims nevertheless to have gained "the same familiarity with disease which the keeper of a menagerie does with the wild beasts he feeds and handles. I there learned the uncertainties of medical observation. The physician is like a watchmaker having charge of watches that he cannot open; he must make the best guess he can, yet it is fair to say that the exploration of the interior of the human body has reached a degree of perfection which was not dreamed of at the time when I was a student."[6]

Holmes's imagery in this brief passage is vivid and telling: diseases, like the wild beasts in a menagerie, become objective realities controllable in the immediacy of the clinic atmosphere, and the familiar watchmaker metaphor is made to apply not to the First Cause of the universe but to the surgeon who explores the universe in microcosm, the body's interior. (The reference to a new degree of "perfection" gained in surgery is a bow to the recent introduction of anesthesia.) Although it would be an injustice to lay too great an emphasis on the reminiscence, one can plainly detect in it the feeling of confidence, even power, over the vagaries of diagnosis that the physician gained from the observational method. It was a confidence all to the good of humanity when wielded in the manner of the outspoken Dr. Holmes, and when prevented, by the leverage of democracy, from becoming the kind of diabolic power portrayed in Hawthorne's Dr. Chillingworth. But romanticists such as Hawthorne and Brown see the darker side of power, even the beneficial powers of medicine, and so their reactions are at times subversive of prevailing attitudes and beliefs. In this way American romance has often served as a corrective to popular, even historical, perspectives.

When the romantic vision falters entirely, however, and fails to record an event of national significance, we are forced to rely on the historical perspective. Such is the case with the cholera epidemics that three times swept portions of the nation in the nineteenth century. It is possible that Hawthorne was moved to write "Lady Eleanore's Mantle," published in 1838, because of the cholera epidemic six years before, especially since both the cholera outbreak and the smallpox epidemic of 1721, which is the premise of his tale, occurred simultaneously in England and America. But the tale makes no reference to cholera and remains closely tied to the smallpox epidemic and the revolutionary "fever" to which the author connects it.

From historical sources we know that another, very different connection was made in the public mind in nineteenth-century America between the highly infectious disease cholera and the "disease" of poverty. As discussed in chapter 4, cholera originated in the poorest, most crime-ridden urban districts; it was principally a disease of the cities and reflected their lack of sanitation, medical help, and proper housing. As is the case with today's urban problems—homelessness, drug addiction, crime, and so forth—government was largely unresponsive until the full force of the threat of contagion to the wider society made itself felt. Only then were measures taken to improve sanitation and reservoirs built to provide the cities with clean water. We look in vain, however, for the American writer who undertook to make the American public "see" the conditions of the urban poor who struggled to maintain a semblance of order amid the widespread social disorder bred by the epidemics. On this subject American literary romanticism all but fails us, with the sole exception of two Edgar Allan Poe tales that offer pictures of epidemic disease but are safely rendered out of an immediate time and place. Bearing in mind, however, the reluctance of American authors to openly address such topics, we might look to such works as Hawthorne's *The Scarlet Letter* (1850) and Herman Melville's *Moby-Dick* (1851) and extrapolate a warning against that national tendency toward association of object with idea that facilitated the linkage of poverty and cholera.

While romanticism was apparently denying the existence of cholera in American cities by turning a blind eye to it, the movement was busily engaging some of the nation's best minds in matters transcendent. More accurately, they were occupied in the formulation of a philosophy, bordering on a religion, that established a clear hierarchy of spirit over matter. One might be tempted to consider this another instance of willful blindness, but so genuine was the impulse behind it and so authentic the texts in which the idea was given form that one dare not risk dismissing transcendentalist philosophy as mere escapism. Stripped of much of its Neoplatonism, it was clearly an attempt to inculcate a value system designed to counter the "thing-ridden" materialism that accompanied the new industrialization. Nor is it at all surprising that transcendentalism began in New England, where Puritan values still echoed in many a public and private voice. Were we able literally to hear those voices today, however, we would hear the racking coughs and the frequent sound of "hemming" (as it was called) that accompanied the effort to clear lungs that were being inexorably consumed by tubercle bacilli. For tuberculosis was also a product of New England; the regional malady spread throughout the country in the nineteenth century, as it did in Europe. Chapter 5 covers the century-plus span during which American writers were made horribly aware (some by the presence of bacilli in their own bodies), as were all Americans, of the toll this epidemical disease was taking. Some writers come close to naming the disease; others suggest its presence by talking about circumstances that in some way parallel the sickness. Almost all the literature contains an economic theme, casting the word *consumption* (used in the nineteenth century to denote tuberculosis) in a somewhat Marxian light and reminding us of the coeval exile of Karl Marx in Brussels, where he produced, with Friedrich Engels, *The Communist Manifesto* (1848), and of Henry Thoreau at Walden. Thoreau's chief complaint—besides the medical one that killed him, TB—was the breakup of the agricultural economy that had been the mainstay of New England and its rapid replacement by an industrial economy. He voices his economic complaint via the same transmutation of ideas employed by most of his contemporaries in attempting to deal with the tuberculosis epidemic—that is, by spiritualizing the dialectic and thus transcending it. Whatever the means of apprehension, nineteenth-century attempts to understand the interrelationships between a nation's economic system and the condition of its people are an outgrowth of the previous century's fascination with the processes of life, death, and disease and evidence a generally rational approach.

= Realism and Communicable Disease =

As the nineteenth century wore on, literary style moved away from romanticism and toward realism, which made it possible to write about subjects previously considered unsuitable, including the subject of illness. Henry James, perhaps the greatest realist in American literature, was finally free to create the heroine he had long wished to see grace the pages of one of his novels. The story of Milly Theale in *The Wings of the Dove* (1902) forms part of the discussion of tuberculosis in chapter 5. Another of James's American heroines, Daisy Miller, also dies of a communicable, though not necessarily epidemic disease. Like Milly Theale, Daisy plays a part in the development of James's international theme of Americans in contact with Europeans. Both young women die in Europe, Milly of what appears to be tuberculosis, Daisy of "Roman fever," or malaria. Since malaria has never been epidemic in America, it falls outside the limits of my discussion, and James's *Daisy Miller* (1879) might be allowed to pass unnoticed except for the important point the author chooses to make about Americans through his heroine's exposure to the disease.

Daisy is not a sickly heroine; she blooms like the flower for which she is named, and with all the innocence the name suggests. That innocence is thrown into doubt, however, because she exhibits a freedom more suited to her native country than to the European scene through which she passes. In Rome she contracts malaria through a reckless act of willful exposure to the disease, an act in which she is encouraged by a European wiser than she to the danger she is courting. In fact, Daisy is betrayed by both Europeans and Americans, none of whom can appreciate the extent of her naïveté. Daisy's imprudent use of her American freedom of action, which results in her death by an infectious disease, suggests a susceptibility—inherent in Americans accustomed only to their own environment—to unfamiliar climates of behavior and opinion as well as of season.

Malaria was, and is, a disease known to both the Old and New Worlds, but in America it had come to be known as the disease of the "newcomer," that is, one who was unseasoned and thus vulnerable to the danger presented by the mix of immune and unimmune populations. One historian of medicine and society in America has said of the susceptibility of the newcomer in a region where malaria threatened, "those blessed with adequate resistance survived."[7] Daisy Miller, inexperienced in the ways of the European environment to which she is exposed, possesses none of the resistance needed for survival there.

Read as a comment on America's faith in its insularity to preserve it from the ills of the Old World, *Daisy Miller* is one of the strongest—and subtlest—statements on infectious disease in American literature. The danger, of course, is in lightly dismissing it as a parable of recklessness; clearly it reflects James's recurrent fear for his countrymen, that through their habit of acting freely and their disregard for, or their ignorance of, the very real dangers of this world, they would participate in their own undoing. One might say that with regard to the danger of contagion intrinsic to relations between America and Europe in the nineteenth century, James advocated inoculation in the form of a greater American awareness of evils to which it had built no resistance.

= Disease and Deviance =

Each chapter in this book deals with an episode of epidemical disease in America that made its way into American literature, either covertly or overtly. The study reveals that the American response to epidemic disease has taken three forms: (1) the panic response of quarantine or separation, which seeks to identify the source and remove it; (2) the denial, or "see no evil" response, which attempts to ignore the presence of disease; and (3) the rational, or scientific response, which seeks to identify the epidemic's source and treat it as well as the disease. All three responses carry the risk of failure. And because romanticism, the dominant literary mode in America, sets itself against rationalism as an alternative point of view—even as an alternative way of knowing—it is within the area of human inadequacy in dealing with epidemics that literature finds its subject matter.

One must be prepared, therefore, to find veiled allusions to the general idea of contagion, and to the specific contagion of epidemical disease, embedded in works that present images of the socially, even criminally, deviant or the sexually unorthodox. Often it is by making the association between these marginalized groups and the perceived threat of contagion they present to the larger society that the American writer is able to move beyond their "otherness" and bring them into focus. Specific literary instances of this are discussed in chapters 3 and 4, but an example taken from film will serve here to illustrate another, invidious use to which the universal fear of epidemic can be put. In the 1950 Elia Kazan film *Panic in the Streets*, contagion operates as the vehicle of a metaphor whose referent is left unspecified.

Panic in the Streets

Late in the 1940s, with World War II barely at an end, the House Un-American Activities Committee began its investigation into Communist influences in American life, with a special interest in the Hollywood film industry. One of the persons named as a Communist in the hearings was filmmaker Elia Kazan, who immediately became fearful of losing the directorial prominence he had recently gained. In Hollywood, where the major product, films, depends heavily on good publicity, the political atmosphere at the time was one of high tension. "Bad press" resulting from governmental denunciations of the industry's leaders as "Communist dupes" (a favorite invective of the committee chairman, Sen. Joseph McCarthy) or worse, could have spelled financial ruin for the film companies. Hollywood chose to police itself; anyone named in the hearings was in danger of being dismissed from the tightly knit industry. While Kazan worriedly awaited his call to testify before the committee in Washington, he began production of a film that appeared in 1950, *Panic in the Streets*. It is the story of an officer in the U.S. Public Health Service (PHS) stationed in New Orleans who almost single-handedly tracks to its source a case of bubonic fever introduced into the city by an illegal alien. Though the victim quickly dies, the disease is passed to a hoodlum-type gambler with whom he comes in contact in his final hours, and so the hunt is on.

None of the film's reviewers suggested that the hero of *Panic in the Streets* could be viewed as engaged in a hunt for the source of another plague, one as deadly—at least in the eyes of the House Un-American Activities Committee—as bubonic fever. Given the political climate of the time, however, the connection seems fairly obvious. Further, in what appears to be a rebuke to those of his colleagues who refused to cooperate with the House committee, Kazan has his young, uniformed PHS doctor meet with resistance from the very people he is trying to save. Their resistance stems from a refusal to recognize the danger they are in and from the fact that he represents to them an authority they distrust. They fail to understand the doctor's argument that their suspicion of the government's motives constitutes a greater threat than the perceived infringement of their freedoms, which must be sacrificed in the interest of tracking down the source of contagion. (Kazan himself confessed to the committee a two-year involvement with the Communist party and offered the names of others involved.) In the end, when the doctor finds his man, the film conveys its most powerful image: the feverishly ill hoodlum attempting to scramble up the rat lines of a moored ship to escape his pursuer. As he pulls himself laboriously hand over hand up the lines, he is stopped by the rat guards, the rounded, metal safety devices on ships dating from the time of the discovery that rats carry plague. Unable to overcome the barrier, the man falls to the water below.

Years later an interviewer asked Kazan if the plague had interested him as a symbol at the time he was making the film. Dismissing the idea, Kazan claimed it was merely "a device, a way of getting into the various sides of the society and the city."[8] Given the threatening nature of his subject and the power of cinematic imagery to convey symbolic messages, the story of a foreign plague that gains entry through America's most vulnerable point, her open ports, seems an obvious reference to the major fear dominating American politics in 1950, the fear of Communists using America's free society to gain entry into the country and overthrow the government. In such a climate the symbolic import of plague can hardly be minimized; it is no mere "device."

For Kazan not to have intended the parallel between plague and communism is impossible to believe.

The problem with such symbolic uses of epidemic disease (aside from their often overly strained connections) is twofold. First, the threat is located outside the United States—or in some cases, outside the mainstream American majority—in a marginalized group. In *Panic in the Streets* the stigma of contagion is attached to illegal aliens and criminals, but it could just as easily be attached to Jews, females, homosexuals, or blacks. The second danger to society in such misleading metaphoric uses of epidemic disease is the dissemination of a distorted view of disease as being like, or even a form of, antisocial behavior. As the story of the yellow fever epidemics in the 1790s makes clear (chapter 3), stigmatizing by association with contagious disease began very early in our national history, and the reading given here of *Edgar Huntly* by Charles Brockden Brown, a survivor of those epidemics, demonstrates the way in which the link between illness and antisocial, or even unorthodox behavior offered an early reinforcement of a view of illness itself as a kind of deviance from a supposed healthy norm. At times of great stress, such as when the nation feels itself threatened or when the government creates a threatening environment, these attitudes surface and individuals often desperately seek to separate the "deviant" sick from the "healthy" norm and to locate themselves firmly within the norm. In this regard, the responsibility of the image creators in society is also twofold: On the one hand, writers, filmmakers, and others are often guilty of making these kinds of damaging associations; on the other hand, they must take responsibility when they fail to acknowledge a true epidemic situation, especially when minorities and marginalized peoples predominate as its invisible victims.

In defense of the artistic community, one can only say that in their blindness to the evils caused by epidemics, as well as to those evils that cause them, American writers and other artists often reflect the attitude of the nation as a whole. It is, however, an attitude that presents a grave danger, for despite their desire to believe in the imperviousness of the New World setting, Americans have proven as vulnerable to true epidemic as any other people. The recent efforts of one segment of society to raise the level of national awareness of the presence of a true epidemic in our midst is the focus of chapter 6, which deals with AIDS. The success of this group, marginalized by the majority, demonstrates how a governmental and societal blindness to this epidemic has been all but turned around by one affected minority determined to gain visibility.

= The 1918 Influenza Epidemic =

As noted earlier, had it not been for Charles Brockden Brown's immediate involvement in the yellow fever epidemics of the 1790s—and his sheer good fortune in having survived—we might not have this first fictional representation of a crucial event in American history. It may be that personal experience of the disease provides the stimulus needed to go against the grain of convention in America and write openly about an epidemic. It is a fact that a number of those who have written about the current AIDS epidemic are themselves infected with the virus. Further, the only literary record of what, until now, was the country's most devastating epidemic, comes from someone who contracted the disease and survived. Had Katherine Anne Porter not been an influenza patient during the 1918 epidemic, the topic would have been as neatly avoided as were the cholera epidemics in the preceding century. Though generally acknowledged by epidemiologists as a pandemic, the influenza epidemic (as it is more commonly known) has left almost no record, literary or historical, in the American consciousness. But it cannot be overlooked in a study of epidemics in America, and since the literary record is too scant to warrant a full chapter, I have chosen to include a brief discussion of it in this introduction.

The End of World War I

A few generations of Americans grew up in a time when it was customary for all normal activity to halt precisely at 11:00 A.M. on 11 November of each year as the nation commemorated what was said to be the exact time when, in 1918, the "war to end all wars" came to an end. It was called Armistice Day (now Veterans Day), and the pleasing symmetry of the commemorative moment happening at the eleventh hour of the eleventh day of the eleventh month helped create for it an indelible mark on the collective mind of most of the world. Certainly in America Armistice Day achieved nationwide commemoration. Not so, however, another historic event of the same year, also with its own mnemonic aid:

> I had a little bird
> And its name was Enza.
> I opened the window
> And in-flew-Enza.[9]

Though the children's rhyme lingers in an abbreviated form—the last two lines are still often used as a rueful explanation for illness—most people are as unaware of the full quatrain as they are of its origins.

Coincident with World War I the world experienced an influenza pandemic that killed, by conservative estimates, some 25 million people, approximately 600,000 of them American citizens. About one-fifth of the world's population had the disease. Add to this figure those who had milder symptoms and were undiagnosed, and one begins to comprehend the scope of

ALLEGHENY COLLEGE LIBRARY

this event. One of the sadder, and socially more damaging effects was that the disease was most lethal to young adults between 20 and 40 years of age, for reasons that have never been clear (though it is readily observable that they would have gained the least immunity from other flus with similar pathology).

It was this high toll of the young that first attracted attention to the disease, for then, as today, influenza was accepted as an inevitable seasonal illness in this part of the world. In 1918 it manifested itself first in March but drew little notice because of the momentous events of the war in Europe, then in its fourth year. Belgium had already succumbed to the German onslaught, and France was pleading for American troops to be sent across the Atlantic to help save it from a similar fate. England knew that the Channel afforded no protection from the determined German forces and joined France in petitioning American president Woodrow Wilson to commit more troops to the French battlefields. Wilson and the American public acceded; in the same month that influenza made its appearance in the United States, 84,000 troops left for Europe, and another 118,000 followed them the next month (Crosby, 18).

The young troops had been together in training camps before embarking, just as other young people of both sexes were working closely together in factories producing war materials and other needed goods, putting in long hours of hard work for the war effort. Both groups were susceptible to influenza by reason of fatigue, stress, and, most of all, mass exposure. Flu swept across North America, entered the ranks, and played havoc with the troops in camps, on board ships, and later in the trenches. It knew no national allegiance and hit both sides of the conflict; German troops fell to this foe more easily than to French forces. European death tolls were extremely high, particularly in Spain, which unwillingly lent its name to the disease. Inexorably it moved on to North Africa, India, the Philippines, and Hawaii—in less than five months.

As the summer came to an end, the epidemic seemed to be subsiding in America. But the nation was sending troops to Europe throughout the period when the epidemic was at its worst there, so that many Americans who did not contract the disease at home got it abroad. At the end of August 1918 the spread of the disease took a new direction. The change occurred in three port areas: Sierra Leone, Africa; Brest, France, a chief disembarkation port for Allied troops; and Boston, Massachusetts, one of the nation's chief embarkation ports. From these three areas the disease moved outward into the rest of the world. This was the worst wave of influenza, made even more dangerous by the heavier congregations of people responding to the need for an even greater war effort. A nearly equal effort went into educating the public about the flu, and posters and warnings appeared everywhere. Everyone was urged to wear gauze masks, and vaccines were administered. By November 1918, when the armistice was signed, the disease was diminishing, but the figures soon started to climb again, and a third wave brought many to their beds before the spring 1919 abatement.

The best guess of today's epidemiologists is that the influenza pandemic began in the United States in March 1918 and was carried to Europe by the troops going "over there" to save our allies. Yet if we think back to the children's rhyme, the name of the free-flying bird—Enza—has a foreign sound, perhaps in an intended allusion to Spain, the supposed country of origin. (Actually, the word *influenza* is Italian.) The bird flies in through the rhymer's window, bringing with it all that its name signifies. Such an interpretation would hardly have been supportive of an all-out war effort on behalf of a portion of the European continent, however, and so it is small wonder that only the last two lines remained as a sort of tag of the whole affair.

And tag it was, not only the rhyme but the epidemic itself, which was perceived as just a tag line to the real event of that year, the war in Europe. Recent studies have shown that even at its height the influenza epidemic in this country never received the journalistic attention it warranted, largely because of America's involvement in the war. Yet the official record reveals that more American soldiers died of the disease than in combat, and that casualties among the civilian population were high enough to suggest a state of siege (Crosby, 206). Still, to this day Americans rarely make any reference to this pestilential outbreak, not even now when they have been made more conscious of epidemics by the AIDS outbreak. "The flu," by which is meant the numerous viral strains that produce varying infections, generally can be avoided now by taking a preventative inoculation made up of those strains expected to infect the general population in a given year. Only the aged, infirm, and chronically ill are considered to be truly at risk. With this as a comforting thought, we skip, as they did in 1918, over the morbidity and mortality figures that make the influenza epidemic real. Only the more senior citizens recall the epidemic from personal experience, and when they do, almost without exception they remember someone young who died that year, not in the war but in a sweat-soaked bed, with a raging fever. Indeed, it is a personal reminiscence of this sort that is the basis of the only piece of American literature to have come out of this epidemic.

"Pale Horse, Pale Rider"

When the influenza epidemic was at its height it was popularly referred to as the Spanish flu, and as "the Spanish lady." "Lady" carried a note of irony, for this lady brought death, as had others of her gender associated in the past with venereal diseases. Although there is no hint of a sexual involvement in Katherine Anne Porter's short story based on her own experience with influenza in 1918, there is a decided undertone of guilt.

The story is of a young newspaperwoman, Miranda Gay, who exhibits none of the clear-eyed cheerfulness her name implies. In the dream with which the story begins she sees the farm where she grew up, with its stables and riding horses. But she also sees a mounted stranger and recognizes him as the same pale rider who was welcomed by her grandfather, great-aunt, a cousin, a dog, and a silver kitten. "Why did they take to him?" she wonders and carefully chooses the horse best suited to outrun this intruder. As he rides beside her she suddenly shouts at him, "I'm not going with you this time—ride on!"[10]

Wakening brings Miranda the same realization that comes with each day's dawning consciousness: "a gong of warning. . . . The war, said the gong" ("Horse," 182). Part of being held captive to the war is the demand for ongoing financial support of the national effort. Miranda feels she cannot afford the cost of a Liberty Bond but is being threatened with dismissal from the paper if she does not sign up. The committee members who visit her at her desk to demand her support keep reminding her that "there's a war on," a realization brought home to her more forcefully when she visits a hospital where soldiers are recovering from war wounds. Ill at ease among them, Miranda decides, "Never again will I come here, this is no sort of thing to be doing" ("Horse," 193).

The extent of Miranda's war involvement is her romance with a young Texas soldier, Adam Barclay, who is temporarily stationed nearby before being sent overseas. Their affair is romantically innocent—even Edenic: Miranda sees her lover Adam as being "like a fine healthy apple" ("Horse," 198). This idyll does not last long, however, for Miranda becomes ill with influenza. Adam nurses her through the first two days of her illness and tells her, when the fever allows her to comprehend, of conditions in the town: "It's as bad as anything can be . . . all the theaters and nearly all the shops and restaurants are closed, and the streets have been full of funerals all day and ambulances all night—" ("Horse," 233). "But not one for me," Miranda responds with the same determination of the girl in her dream, and she is correct, for Adam's attentions, followed by good medical care at a local hospital, pull her through. Adam returns to camp and dies of influenza before he is shipped overseas.

The news of Adam's death does not reach Miranda for a month, during which time she is fighting for her own life. Once recovered, and even before learning of her lover's death, she has ceased to rejoice in her returning health. While caught up in the fevered sleep that comes with the disease she had felt herself happier among the dead; when she awakes, to celebrations of the armistice, she feels herself "an alien who does not like the country in which he finds himself" ("Horse," 257). She is further alienated by the knowledge of Adam's death and leaves the hospital with a feeling of emptiness and a dread of the lonely years that stretch ahead of her: "No more war, no more plague, only the dazed silence that follows the ceasing of the heavy guns;

noiseless houses with the shades drawn, empty streets, the dead cold light of tomorrow. Now there would be time for everything" ("Horse," 264). Time enough for the guilt that Miranda feels, and that Porter herself once admitted to her biographer.[11]

So closely associated were the war and the influenza epidemic that Americans were unable to concentrate on the two separately. Just as Miranda Gay feels guilty for having survived the disease and for having infected another—and someone who, unlike her, was willing to support the war effort to the fullest—Americans on the home front appear to have felt guilty for making too much of the disease that was striking them down. Porter's reference to time—"Now there would be time for everything"—is also significant, for Americans simply did not have time enough to give the necessary attention to a full-blown epidemic while in the midst of war. For many who suffered the loss of loved ones but had no time to mourn while the war still demanded all their attention, and for those who hurried their own recovery, not allowing sufficient time for the necessary psychological and physiological healing, there must surely have been a sense of unfinished business connected to the epidemic. "Now there would be time for everything" also reminds one of the youthfulness of so many of the victims, robbed of precious time, and of the brevity of the epidemic as well as the brevity of the illness itself. People became ill and either recovered or died all in a matter of a month—just about as long as some love affairs or marriages last in a time of war. On balance, then, "Pale Horse, Pale Rider," by its own brevity, its intermingling of war and epidemic, and its acknowledgment of feelings of guilt, is as good a literary record as one could wish of an event that has otherwise passed into history all but unnoted.

Katherine Anne Porter provided the world with what one might call a firsthand report of the influenza epidemic in the United States. A more recent portrayal of small-town America caught in the grip of this pestilence is Horton Foote's 1979 drama, *1918*. Part of a nine-play cycle entitled *The Orphans' Home Cycle* (the title is based on a Marianne Moore poem), *1918* focuses on a Texas family caught up in the fast-spreading, and even faster killing, disease believed by many in the small town to be "part of what they call germ warfare" being waged against America by Germany.[12] Two generations of one family are united by their common experience of sickness and death, a drama that plays out on the small-town level while in the background the global conflict, World War I, draws to a close. Foote's dramatic achievement is his ability to make the epidemic and its devastating personal effects dwarf the international conflict so that momentarily we are made to care more for the death by influenza of a single child than for all the war dead lying in far-off fields or hospitals.

Because of the double focus of this volume on historical as well as literary records not all episodes of epidemical disease in the United States have been

treated equally, and some are not even touched on if they received no direct
literary representations. Poliomyelitis was epidemic in the United States on
at least three occasions in the twentieth century and affected a great many
people, including one who became the nation's president. But it left no literary
record, no product of the artistic imagination by which we might gauge the
influence of this epidemic on the collective imagination of the people afflicted
or otherwise forced to deal with it. Medical history is insufficient evidence for
determining the full effect of an epidemical devastation of a people, and the
interpretation of that history is often best aided by the creative works that
arise from it. An understanding of the culture from which the creative work
derives is the final requisite, of course, but the subtleties of the underlying
structures that shape thought can be elusive. Thought patterns about disease
may not even manifest themselves in imaginative literature and have often
remained in the area of medical arts, a case in point being the difference
of opinion over the efficacy of live or killed vaccine as a preventative of
poliomyelitis.

The question (pertinent also to flu vaccines) involves the difference
between injecting, as in the Sabin vaccine, a live polio virus specially bred to
provide immunity but not infection, and injecting an actual polio virus that
has been chemically killed to achieve the same effect, as in the Salk vaccine.
Differences in the degree and duration of immunity offered by these two
methods may have been the sole determining medical factor in the movement
away from the Salk vaccine, but an underlying fear of the actual polio virus—
even though killed—seems to have played at least an equal part. Seeking to
allay this fear, Jonas Salk has insisted that "immunity can be divorced from
infectivity," by which he means that the immunizing agent need not be viable
to prove effective but should be genuinely characteristic of the disease against
which it protects.[13] The notion seems to contradict, however, the thought
patterns of Americans, who value immunity from evil and believe it is possible
to remain free of its infection. Is this notion embedded in the national psyche?
Perhaps, though more likely it has its roots in the Judeo-Christian mythos of
humankind's "infection" as a result of Adam's fall. In the New World Garden
of the modern mythos, the American dream was that infection might be
avoided entirely and immunity gained through virtue, science, and distance
from the source of evil—Europe.

2

The Pathology of Revolution

IN 1721 BOSTON EXPERIENCED THE WORST EPIDEMIC OF SMALL-
pox in its history. This dreaded disease, which afflicted peoples throughout
the world, had a long history but acquired its name late in the fifteenth
century when the great pox, syphilis, with which it was associated, swept
through Europe. The coincidence of the eruption of syphilis in Europe with
explorations into the regions of the New World gave rise to the medical
chauvinism that underlies ascriptions of epidemical diseases to specific nations. Hence the sixteenth-century treatise by Girolamo Fracastoro names the
disease "syphilis" but offers as an alternative, *morbus Gallicus*, the "French
disease." It was Fracastoro who linked together measles, syphilis, and smallpox, declaring them contagious diseases capable of being spread by direct
person-to-person contact or through intermediate agents such as clothing,
bedding, and so forth.

Sailors had always been suspect in these matters, and with good reason.
Trade routes followed the routes of conquest, and just as the Roman army
returned victorious from its assault on the Parthians in A.D. 164 but carrying

away smallpox from that central Asian empire, so the disease reached the West Indies only about 15 years after Columbus made his initial voyage to the New World. The Spaniards brought smallpox to Mexico and to Central and South America, so that it became known in parts of Europe as the Spanish pox; in England, once it was distinguished from syphilis, it was no longer called the French pox (that name being reserved for the venereal disease) but variola, the "small pox." Without the unintended biological weapon of smallpox, which their acquired immunity allowed them to wield with impunity, the Spaniards would have faced a more formidable enemy in the Indian populations they sought to conquer. Some historians who believe the Amerindians to have been the source of the European plague of syphilis view smallpox as the European revenge.[1]

It is (or was, since smallpox was officially declared eradicated by the World Health Organization [WHO] in 1979) a strange disease. Viral in nature, smallpox caused fever and the malaise generally associated with fever. With these symptoms came ulcerous bodily eruptions—worst on the face, hands, and feet—that left permanent disfigurement. Less well-known but frequent impairments were blindness and crippling. Mortality rates during a smallpox epidemic were extremely high, largely because the first to succumb to the disease were children who had not been previously exposed and who thus had no immunity. The disease spread rapidly among this population, exacting a severe toll. If no previous epidemic had occurred within the lifetime of the affected population, adults too had no immunity and were as susceptible as children. The English historian Thomas Macaulay wrote of the disease "filling the churchyards with corpses," and "tormenting with constant fears all whom it had not yet stricken." Describing the disfigurement of its survivors, Macaulay claimed smallpox left the hideous traces of its power, turning the babe into a changeling at which the mother shuddered, and making the eyes and cheeks of the betrothed maiden objects of horror to the lover.[2] Macaulay's emotionally charged description portends the romanticism of Nathaniel Hawthorne's tale of the epidemic in colonial Boston; such were the horrors of this disease that a historian's account could readily suggest a romanticist's art.

Smallpox was a viral disease. In the course of this study we shall encounter other viruses, and it is important to distinguish clearly between diseases caused by bacterial and viral infection. Despite their single-cell state and their multiplication by simple division, bacteria are fairly complex microorganisms that occur in three main forms, spherical (cocci), rod-shaped (bacilli), and spiral (spirilla). Wine would not be possible except for the fermentation of bacteria, nor would renewed amounts of nitrogen plant foods occur in soil without the presence of bacteria. But bacteria also live in human and animal soft tissue, blood, and bones, where they feed off their host in a parasitical way and poison it with their waste, causing disease. The list of these diseases is long and includes some of the most dreaded among humankind: tuberculosis, typhoid fever, syphilis, leprosy, anthrax, tetanus, whooping cough, diptheria, scarlet fever, gonorrhea, bubonic plague, and pneumonia. Fortunately, bacteria can be grown outside host bodies so that their precise nature, and their weaknesses, can be determined. They are vulnerable to a wide range of chemical substances that either inhibit their growth or destroy them; among the more widely known antibiotics are penicillin, streptomycin, and tetracycline.

Viruses, however, are another matter. Like bacteria, they are microorganisms, but except under certain laboratory conditions, they do not reproduce outside living cells. This characteristic has made their study very difficult, since it is not always possible to distinguish clearly between their properties and those of the host cell. Among the diseases they cause are poliomyelitis, measles, chicken pox, mumps, smallpox, rabies, dengue and yellow fever, some types of influenza and pneumonia, the common cold, and AIDS. Because of the difficulty in studying these organisms, there is no specific drug treatment for most viral diseases. But many of them provide immunity against further attacks of the same disease, so vaccines have been developed that, when injected into the body, develop a similar immunity. Another problem with viruses is that they are capable of transforming cells by altering genetic information; they can mutate so rapidly that, as with influenzas, it is necessary to regularly revise the vaccine substances used against them. A further complication has come to light through the relatively recent recognition of another category of slow-acting viruses, such as HIV-1, the virus that causes AIDS. Retroviruses, which implant themselves in cells and cause disease much later, are responsible for progressive and generally fatal diseases, against which there are no vaccines.

Smallpox accompanied many of the colonists on their voyage to the New World, robbing some of the desired end of their journey but affording others a degree of immunity that took them safely through the earliest outbreaks of the disease in New England. When the New World natives were exposed to the disease for the first time, they died in great numbers while the English, immunized by previous exposure, remained largely unaffected, a medical phenomenon that was seen by the colonists as a sign of God's preferment of the settlers and as a judgment on the natives. Throughout the seventeenth century there were scattered outbreaks in the colonies, some more serious than others, but on the whole the colonists were more protected than victimized by them, for each succeeding generation of survivors acquired an immunity to further outbreaks.

Significantly, the first medical treatise by an American was occasioned by a smallpox outbreak in 1677. Its author was the Rev. Thomas Thacher, minister to South Church in Boston. Like Cotton Mather, whose stand on smallpox inoculation became a matter of no small importance, the Rev. Thacher was deeply concerned for his congregation; but unlike Mather, he was a skilled doctor, though he had no physician's license. With material culled from the writings of the famous English physician Thomas Sydenham,

Thacher wrote *A Brief Rule to guide the Common-People of New-England, How to order themselves and theirs in the Small Pocks, or Measels* and posted it on the door of South Church for all to read.

Near the end of the century a smallpox outbreak of truly epidemic proportions raged through Canada, into New England, and as far south as New York. In 1690 the epidemic struck Salem, Massachusetts; two years later it may have seemed to inhabitants of that community a rehearsal for the "epidemic" of witchcraft that followed. Indeed, as the colonists entered the eighteenth century, some of those who had been involved in the witchcraft epidemic of 1692 found themselves once again caught up in an epidemical fever when smallpox ravaged Boston in 1721. One of these, Cotton Mather, who defended the Salem trials in his *Wonders of the Invisible World* (1693), took as firm a hand with the disease as he had with the witches.

= Cotton Mather and Inoculation =

Cotton Mather, third-generation Puritan (second-generation in the New World) and minister to the congregation of North Church in Boston, was not a man to be easily cowed by outbreaks of either illness or witchcraft. Nor was he easily swayed by public opinion; though he took a hard line on the matter of witches, he stubbornly refused to accept the popular notion of spectral evidence—testimony that ill-doing had been wrought by the specters, or apparitions, of those accused of witchcraft. Spectral evidence was admissible in the courts of Old and New England. Mather, however, projected yet another court, functioning in the realm of the invisible, and feared that too vigorous an exercise of authority against individuals accused of spectrally wreaking harm on their neighbors might obtain for "the devils" in the courts of the invisible world, "a license to proceed unto most hideous desolations."[3]

This absolute faith in the coexistence of two realms, visible and invisible, stood Mather in good stead when dealing with the invisible causes of a very apparent disease. The man was no stranger to this disease, for the epidemic that swept through New England in 1713 did not spare Mather's family despite his ministerial position: three of his children and a housemaid died within a month. But when it returned in 1721 his firm resolve suggests that he had armed himself to do battle with this visitant from the invisible realm.

The pox made its appearance in April, and by September the *Boston Gazette*, eager to minimize its effect, incorrectly reported 110 deaths and more than 1,500 survivors. The emphasis on survivors was meant to distinguish the outcome of epidemical disease in the New World from the heavy death toll exacted by similar diseases in Europe. But by the following spring it was clear that, in a total population of nearly 11,000, there had been in the neighborhood of 6,000 cases, of which nearly 1,000 were fatal.[4] These were unusually high figures given the scant two decades that had elapsed since the last major epidemic, but in those decades a large number of children had been born who had no immunity. The figures suggest not only the virulency of the siege but the urgency of the situation, which seemed to demand remedy.

No effective treatment was available for the 6,000 citizens of Boston who fell victim, nor was there much in the way of prevention for the remaining 5,000. The usual measures were to scrutinize ships seeking entry to the harbor (in 1721 it was a ship from Salt Tortuga that brought the disease) so that any persons ill from infectious disease might be removed to the public hospital built for this purpose on an island in the harbor. When it became apparent that, once again, a ship had brought infection to the city, houses were searched for sick persons and black males were put to work cleaning the streets. The practice of hiring blacks for this purpose was common, for reasons that will soon become evident. As the disease gripped the entire city, those who could fled to safer precincts, leaving those who could not to care for themselves as best they might.

These latter, "Miserables neglected and perishing in Sickness," became the object of Cotton Mather's concern. Many of them were his parishioners, and he feared for the condition of their bodies as he did for their souls. This care brought him to their bedsides for prayer, inevitably a place of danger to himself as well as to his own family. Having lost three children in the previous epidemic, he felt the same fate hanging over the two children born subsequently, who were unprotected by an acquired immunity. Following the usual practice in Puritan New England, Mather declared days of prayer and fasting and preached on the need to rid the community of sin to dispel the pestilential scourge. But Mather was prepared to go beyond these ecclesiastical measures and to take a direct hand in the matter.

He was a man who had long been interested in science; he had been elected to the Royal Society of London in 1713 largely on the strength of his serious interest in medicine and the series of New World *Curiosa Americana* (1712–24) that he began sending to London in 1712. After the smallpox epidemic, which brought him to prominence in the field of medicine, he began work on *The Angel of Bethesda* a medical work that was not published in his lifetime. Here he offered advice on the care of the body so closely linked to pastoral concerns that it firmly established his preeminence among the ministerial physicians of New England. These pastor-physicians, as they have been called, owed their dual calling to the oppression that denied dissenters access to ministerial positions in the established Church of England. Such young men pursued theological studies but prudently added anatomy courses that would make them eligible for medical careers. When they came to America they brought, along with their theological calling, sorely needed medical skills. Once removed from access to medical information, however, many pastor-physicians were forced to rely heavily on methods of treatment learned in earlier years; many used popular folk remedies as well. Not so Cotton Mather, whose scientific curiosity never waned and who more and more centered his attention, because of the dire nature of the disease, on smallpox. Sydenham's seventeenth-century observations on the disease had greatly intrigued Mather, who considered himself an empiricist, that is, one who depends upon facts rather than speculation. He readily embraced the knowledge of animalcules introduced through the use of microscopes. Animalcules, or germs, as they were later known, became visible to the human eye for the first time in the seventeenth century, and empirical scientists recognized in them a remote cause of illness. The theory of external disease causation—etiology—departed from the earlier belief that disease was internally caused—pathology.

The importance of Mather's acceptance of etiological, or external, sources as the cause of illness and disease should not be overlooked: despite his religious faith he was able to acknowledge that illness is not necessarily a punishment from God, and that contagious disease need not be merely endured if something can be done to avert the entry into the body of a disease-bearing organism. Still, a great leap of medical faith was needed to move from that level of awareness to the seemingly contradictory idea that a small amount of the disease-bearing organism might be deliberately introduced into a healthy body to ensure its continued health. It is not an easy concept to assimilate even now, but in his eagerness to deal with the evil of smallpox Mather proved himself willing to accept information from sources other than those who were schooled and learned in medicine.

In June 1721, while the epidemic was gathering force in the city, Mather addressed a letter to the local physicians praising a "Wonderful Practice" of which he recently had learned. The practice of inoculation was known in Africa, India, and the Orient and was the reason blacks in the colonies were pressed into service for street cleaning during epidemics: they appeared to have a natural immunity to the disease. In fact, the practice of inoculation was first described to Mather in 1714 by a black servant, Onesimus, who assured him that he himself had been so immunized, as were most of his people. (It should be remembered that, in inoculation, pus or scab matter from an infected person was introduced into the body of a well person who, once infected, could transmit the disease; in vaccination, developed by Dr. Edward Jenner in 1796, the cowpox virus is injected, which provides protection from smallpox. A vaccinated person cannot transmit the virus.) Mather embraced this news of the folk practice joyously, especially when, a few months later, he read the account of Dr. John Woodward, a London physician, who described inoculations in Constantinople. In 1718 Lady Mary Wortley Montagu published an eyewitness report of the Constantinople inoculations; Mather was ready to see the practice begun in Boston.

His eagerness did not prevent him from realizing that the practice described by an ignorant black servant was hardly likely to find converts among the physicians of Boston. So to his letter he added a detailed account of what he had read in the *Transactions*: for at least 40 years doctors in Constantinople had taken from young persons stricken by the disease infected matter that was entered into the blood of healthy persons by means of several small cuts in the arm. When the inevitable fever and pustules broke out, the patient spent only a few days in bed and was soon well, with but a small number of "pock" marks to show that he had been infected.

Mather found a ready convert to this practice in Dr. Zabdiel Boylston, who, though he lacked a medical degree, had a reputation for bold and daring feats of medicine (Silverman, 340). In fact, Boylston's reputation had brought him too much publicity for one whose title of "Doctor" was merely honorary and was based on his academic training. Although it was common practice for such individuals to practice medicine in America—even after the Revolution, because of the scarcity of medical doctors—they were expected to bow to the superior knowledge of the physicians. As shall be seen, Boylston failed to do so. By June 1721 Boylston was ready, with Mather's encouragement, to begin; his first inoculees were a black male servant, a small black child, and— bravely—his own son, aged six years. All three experiments went well, and Boylston prepared to teach the practice to other doctors. (There was clearly a danger in a poorly administered inoculation: Jonathan Edwards, the philosopher and Puritan orator, died in 1758 of a smallpox inoculation that went wrong.) The reaction of the people of Boston, however, was to accuse the doctor of spreading the disease by infecting healthy individuals. Initially, Mather was exonerated as one who meant to do good, though in a mistaken fashion. Inoculations were soon forbidden by the selectmen of the city.

If the reaction of the local government seems shortsighted, one need only consider what inoculation involves, and how dreadful it would have seemed in the eighteenth century to those who had no concept of the ability of the "small dose" to ward off the large dose of infection. As the summer of 1721 wore on and cases of smallpox continued to mount, news came from abroad that bubonic plague had struck in France and parts of the Mediterranean region. Dr. Boylston was not to be restrained further, and against express orders, he continued to inoculate. Mather, meanwhile, continued to write on the subject and offered the opinion, novel in his day, that the disease might be caused by live creatures observable through a microscope. As his most recent biographer has said, this speculation was a tremendous advance toward the germ theory of disease (Silverman, 344); it is also wholly consistent with the Puritan minister's absolute faith in the existence of spiritual entities that are not observable, even with the aid of a microscope.

A new contestant now entered the fray, a Boston newspaper destined to make an impact not only on its time but on American literature. The paper, the *New-England Courant*, was owned and printed by one James Franklin, whose younger brother Benjamin was in his employ. The *Courant* seemed to have but one object—to flout authority, whether governmental or ecclesiastical. It took special delight in tweaking the noses of such Puritan divines as Cotton Mather, whose public espousal of a forbidden practice now offered the newspaper a wonderful opportunity to do just that in the guise of defending the public order. By providing a forum for the only doctor in Boston who actually possessed a medical degree, Dr. William Douglass, the *Courant* helped mobilize the city against inoculation (Silverman, 345). Douglass was quite serious in his opposition, but the newspaper simply saw the controversy as a chance to publicly ridicule the stalwart Mather.

=   The "Silence Dogood" Letters   =

When young Benjamin Franklin observed the glee with which the people of Boston received writers who attacked the educated clergy, he was "excited" to join them, as he says in his *Autobiography* (1793). Thus began the "Silence Dogood" series of letters that young Franklin originally submitted without even his brother knowing whose work they were. The first letter appeared in April 1722, a year after the outbreak of Boston's worst smallpox epidemic. By then the epidemic had passed, and Franklin, keen to the necessity of keeping the newspaper current, made no reference to the inoculation controversy. Nevertheless, his choice of pseudonym, "Dogood," and of persona—the landlady of the town's minister—could not help but direct attention toward Cotton Mather, author of *Bonifacius* (1710), or "Essays to Do Good." "Silence" may have been derived from Mather's sermon of September 1721 entitled "Silentiarius." The theme of the sermon was, "Our God is never more *Praised* than by our *silence*." If this sermon was in fact the source for Franklin's female persona, it was a cruel joke, for Mather had preached the sermon as a sign of his own resignation before God at the death of yet another of his children (Silverman, 348).

    The youthful Franklin, heady with his own "wit," would not have hesitated at such cruelty if he had thought it would help reduce the haughtiness of the clergy, especially the renowned Mather, for the *Courant* took the part of the common people against those who considered themselves their betters. And true to form, the most famous of the Silence Dogood letters, the dream vision in which Silence is conducted to the great hall of Learning (Harvard College), brought a rejoinder from Cotton Mather's son Samuel, a Harvard student, in which he demonstrated that his own erudition was greater than that of the letter writer.[5] Still, the *Courant*'s anti-intellectualism did not prevent it from featuring the opinions of Dr. William Douglass, who was obviously a learned doctor. It would appear, then, that the local citizenry had little trouble choosing, between the authority of theology or of medicine, the greater foe.

    What the *Courant* failed to realize, however, was the tremendous step forward in empirical knowledge that Cotton Mather made in adopting the idea of inoculation. Not even an attempted assassination—by means of a grenade thrown through a window of his house and bearing the inscription,

"Cotton Mather, You Dog, Dam you; I'l inoculate you with this, with a Pox to you"—could dissuade this minister of God from his firm belief that it was not God's will for individuals to die when there was a means of saving them (Silverman, 350). Gradually he was able to convince other members of the clergy, who then also became objects of ridicule. Indeed, as the epidemic year wore on, writers in the *Courant* began to assume a "holier than thou" attitude toward the inoculating pastor-physicians, accusing them not only of infecting those who were healthy but of usurping the authority of God by deliberately introducing into the community what was His province to inflict as He saw fit—disease.[6]

Behind this argument is both the idea of the covenanted community and the principal form by which the idea had been kept alive in New England for three generations—the jeremiad, a genre of sermon named for the Old Testament prophet Jeremiah, whose warnings to the Israelites invariably included a recital of the afflictions God had allowed to fall upon his chosen people for their shortcomings. Widely employed in England by the dissenting clergy, the jeremiad became in America a public ritual by means of which the New England ministers joined their criticism of the Puritan communities with their urgings toward spiritual renewal.[7] It was far more than a revivalist ritual—made familiar in this country later by traveling evangelists—because the concern of the Puritan clergy was for both the spiritual and social order of the covenanted community. The subject of the jeremiad was nothing less than the political body of believers represented by their church affiliation.

The Puritan church was made up of individuals who had covenanted with God and with each other in voluntary, purposeful union, just as the people of Abraham had covenanted together and with Jehovah. Therefore, the church body, which was considered to be the bride of Christ, had to be kept spiritually and physically whole, free of anything that would violate its soundness and purity. Because the New England Puritans had sacrificed so much for the sake of a pure church, contagion, whether of disease or ideas, was perceived as a constant threat to the Puritan body politic. One can see how strong was the fear of contagious ideas merely by considering the long-standing Puritan animosity toward Quakers. Like witchcraft, the Quaker doctrine was anathema to the Puritans. But their physical presence in the community was even worse, and not solely because they refused to acknowledge the authority of the ministry: the communication of their beliefs represented an infection spread through the Puritan community.

Prior to the 1721 outbreak of the disease, smallpox epidemics had been looked upon as one of the scourges by which God recalled his wanton people. Since the afflictions of God were always presented by the clergy as corrective, the argument used by Mather's detractors—that by advocating inoculation the minister was interfering with God's correction of his children and thwarting the judgment of heaven upon those who would otherwise be stricken—turned back on Mather the rhetoric by which for so long the ministry, including

Cotton and his father, Increase, had chastened God's children (Miller, 349). The rhetorical ground of the jeremiad was thus shifted away from its earlier millennial cast and turned in a new and democratic direction.

To appreciate the importance of this shift it is necessary to recall that the underpinning of the jeremiad was the allegorical application of the biblical exodus of the Israelites to the Puritan exodus out of Anglican England. The wilderness experience of the people chosen by Jehovah, and the subsequent record of their relationships with other peoples, was a history of falling out of covenant with Jehovah, necessitating the role of the prophets exemplified by Jeremiah. Part of the allegorical interpretation of the Puritan errand into the New World wilderness was the role of the ministry in watching for signs of a similar dereliction. When the *Courant* turned against the clergy in 1721 and accused it (in the person of Cotton Mather) of deserting its duty, the charge acquired a degree of combined virtue and patriotism that only the jeremiad tradition could lend. As if this were not enough, the newspaper also ridiculed the clergy for earlier instances of ministerial misjudgment in times of social upheaval. The *Courant*'s editor, James Franklin, with obvious reference to Cotton Mather's earlier endorsement of the general condemnation of Salem's "witches," pointed to this new medical theory as the latest form of ministerial error. Nor was this controversy subject matter for the editor alone; encouraged by the newspaper's stand, its readers provided a steady supply of letters and articles on the inoculation question throughout the fall and winter of 1721, most of them anti-inoculation and anti-clergy.

Obviously Benjamin Franklin spoke for many New Englanders who had tired of their clergymen and of the imperious, authoritarian manner with which the clergy treated them. It was a manner akin to that of their English rulers, and of those sent from England to govern their colonies. One of the latter was Gov. Samuel Shute. Appointed governor of Boston by George I, Shute had sought, a month before the smallpox outbreak, a licensing act by which to gain control of newspapers that fomented factionalism (such as the *Courant* proved to be). Yet Shute was a man Cotton Mather admired to the point of flattery. No wonder that readers of the *Courant* lumped the Puritan ministers together with the civil authorities under whom they chafed, and that they were willing to use the inoculation controversy against them.

Mather's embrace of the inoculation theory has been questioned and evaluated in different ways by scholars. Perry Miller's judgment seems unkind but may simply be born of a need to support his belief in the jeremiad as a religious exercise and ordering principle in the declining years of Puritanism in America. For him the problem is that Mather, by promulgating inoculation, went against the principle of the jeremiad, which was to call for spiritual reform, not medical treatment, in the face of apparent divine wrath. Miller sees Mather as grasping at whatever straws of the coming Enlightenment he could to prove his own wisdom in a desperate attempt to maintain the authority of the ministry over the body and soul of the believer (Miller, 345).

Kenneth Silverman ascribes more generous motives to Mather and excuses his zeal on the ground that he was not a trained physician but a minister moved by compassion (Silverman, 361). He points to the vindication of Mather's position by the Royal Society in London, which took seriously his essay on smallpox and the effectiveness of inoculation. (Inoculation was introduced in England in 1721, the same year it was tried in Boston, but it did not become a widespread practice until the 1740s.) An earlier critic, Dr. Oliver Wendell Holmes, put it succinctly when he urged that Mather's record in the smallpox controversy be set against the same divine's recommendation that witches be searched for marks and subjected to the water ordeal. For the purposes of this investigation, however, it is not the judgments of scholars and historians that really matter; what counts is the perception of Mather's contemporaries, even—perhaps especially—that of the brash youth Benjamin Franklin.

Though wrongheaded in his condemnation of inoculation, in this controversy Franklin represents, as he does in his later *Autobiography*, the spirit of the new nation, which expressed itself in 1722 by taking convenient aim at the declining Puritan ministry. Years later Franklin had reason to bitterly regret his stance on inoculation when his uninoculated four-year-old son died in a Philadelphia epidemic. In Boston in 1721, however, the power of the ministry had to be destroyed, by whatever means, on behalf of younger Americans with more democratic impulses. The deference that earlier had been directed toward the ministry could not just be diverted into new channels; the authority of the pulpit had to be completely undermined. Franklin, behind whose humor lurked the anger he harbored against all those, including his brother James, who would play the master, pilloried the ministers of Boston, especially the influential Mathers, and was no less effective for his apparent flippancy. The boldness of the *Courant* staff in tackling authority presaged the power of collective bargaining instituted by the printers of New York in 1778, when they were the first group in the newly independent nation to successfully negotiate pay increases. This movement toward a collective use of power, occurring early in our national history, is one of the significant instances of democratic power arising out of the epidemics that have occurred in the United States.

As early as the 1730s the New England ministry was rapidly losing much of its power, thanks in part to the efforts of the Franklin brothers, who seized the opportunity of the smallpox epidemic to help diminish it. The struggle for democratic rights, led by the *New-England Courant*, in the inoculation controversy was like an opportunistic infection: it took advantage of an already weakened (immune) system to gain a position of power. Smallpox was the primary infection, but the rebelliousness that the *Courant* brought to the controversy was evidence of a larger social and political dis-ease. Had Cotton Mather been proven correct in his endorsement of inoculation, it would have revived his waning power, something the *New-England Courant* and its subscribers saw as a greater ill than smallpox.

═ "Lady Eleanore's Mantle" ═

The idea of two ills raging through Boston in 1721, smallpox and social unrest of the kind that engenders revolutionary fever, underlies Nathaniel Hawthorne's somewhat muddled allegory of the epidemic, "Lady Eleanore's Mantle." The story was published in 1838 and is one of the tales based on colonial history through which Hawthorne attempted to establish himself as an *American* writer. The problem with trying to read the allegory "correctly," that is (in the language of allegorical interpretation), to apprehend its moral meaning, is the same problem encountered often in reading Hawthorne: one runs up against his sense of psychological division, rooted in his awareness of himself as an inheritor of both Puritan order and revolutionary disorder. Any attempt by the second of these forces to overcome the first would have to be, according to the moral concepts that ruled Hawthorne's psyche, grounded in a kind of pride and arrogance. This is why one's impressions of Robin Molineux, in "My Kinsman, Major Molineux" (1832), are so mixed: while admiring his persistence in seeking his kinsman, the means to his fortune, in colonial Boston, we are shocked by the alacrity with which Robin chooses to side against the major when that fortune is no longer attainable. This youth's "shrewdness," to which Hawthorne repeatedly calls our attention, is but a by-product of the pride of name he has demonstrated at every encounter in the search for his erstwhile politically powerful kinsman. Hawthorne further reveals his ambivalence about the means (though never the end itself) by which the colonies gained their independence when he moves us to great pity at the sight of Robin's tormented kinsman: tarred and feathered, he has been made the object of a minor revolution that prefigures the greater one to come. In "Lady Eleanore's Mantle" Hawthorne also presents a prefiguration of the Revolution but undercuts the full force of its political potential by cloaking it in an anticontagionist rite of repentance and purification.

As Hawthorne recounts the smallpox epidemic of 1721, the disease is probably, though not certainly, imported into the Massachusetts Bay area not by some ignoble seaman off a merchant ship but by "a young lady of rank and fortune arrived from England," Lady Eleanore Rochcliffe.[8] The young woman, recently orphaned, has arrived in the colony to claim the protection of her guardian, Gov. Samuel Shute (the same Gov. Shute who demanded the licensing of newspapers in Boston). The Lady Eleanore, however, is possessed of a "harsh, unyielding pride," and "it seemed due from Providence that pride so sinful should be followed by as severe a retribution" ("Mantle," 273–74). Thus is the stage set for what appears to be a predictable moral tale, complicated only by the presence in the colony of Jervase Helwyse, a young man who, having met the Lady Eleanore in London, loves her distractedly but whose affection she dismisses as of no consequence. At the lady's arrival in the colony, Helwyse, who gives every indication of being deranged by his hopeless love, abases himself by offering his own prostrate body as a carpet for her to step on as she leaves her carriage. Granting him the "favor," she places her foot on his back as she extends her hand to the governor, "and never, surely, was there an apter emblem of aristocracy and hereditary pride, trampling on human sympathies and the kindred of nature, than these two figures presented at that moment," Hawthorne says ("Mantle," 276).

At the governor's ball given to welcome her, Lady Eleanore's beauty is set off by the splendor of an embroidered mantle, which Hawthorne invests with that hint of magical quality peculiar to his invention. The lady displays, however, a fevered eye and flushed countenance as well as an air of languor mixed with her usual hauteur. Disdaining the champagne served as refreshment, she is suddenly presented by the love-maddened Helwyse with a wine-filled silver goblet that he describes as "holy." He begs her to drink of it and then to pass the goblet among the guests as a symbolic gesture that she has not sought to withdraw herself "from the chain of human sympathies" ("Mantle," 280). When she refuses, he breaks out with another request, that she throw off the mantle from her shoulders. Though he refers to it as "accursed," she scorns him and draws the embroidered piece more tightly to her. With a final word, a seemingly knowing allusion to the alteration of her features that is to come, Helwyse allows himself to be forcibly ejected from the Province House ball.

Watching from a distance in the great ballroom is a Dr. Clarke; he eyes Lady Eleanore with "knowing sagacity" and then speaks privately to her protector, the governor, who quickly terminates the ball. Within days smallpox ravages the city. Hawthorne describes it as "distinguished by a peculiar virulence, insomuch that it has left its traces . . . on the history of the country, the affairs of which were thrown into confusion by its ravages" ("Mantle," 282). The disease begins first among the highly positioned inhabitants of the colony, those who had been welcomed to the governor's ball, from whence it spreads throughout all levels of the stricken society, making "brethren" of all.

The apparent cause of this misery, the Lady Eleanore, lies closeted in her room at the Province House, but Jervase Helwyse forces his way past the governor in an effort to see her. Bearing aloft a red banner of the type used to signal a house in which the plague has struck, Helwyse ascends the stair to her room. As he shakes the flag he cries out that Death and Pestilence will walk the streets that night, and that he must march before them with the banner. At the door of the sickroom Helwyse finds Dr. Clarke, who denounces the Lady Eleanore to him as the bearer to "our shores" of the pestilence and death that, he claims, she has released from the folds of her mantle. Yet he allows Helwyse to enter. Expecting to find her usual beauty, Helwyse is horrified at the "[h]eap of diseased mortality" that he finds behind the bed curtains. The lady acknowledges that she is the cause of the epidemic, because "I wrapped myself in PRIDE as in a MANTLE, and scorned the sympathies of nature" ("Mantle," 287).

To this point Hawthorne seems to have worked out his allegory nicely, using Pride, the first of the deadly sins as they were ordered in the Middle Ages, as the progenitor of pestilence and death. But in the story's final paragraph Hawthorne muddies the waters by presenting one of those processional scenes out of Edmund Spenser's *The Faerie Queene*, a sixteenth-century allegory to which Hawthorne remained attached throughout his life. It is a torchlight procession, much like the one in "My Kinsman, Major Molineux," but in place of a live victim of scorn this processional has at its center the figure of a woman wrapped in a mantle. Leading the procession and waving the red flag of pestilence is Jervase Helwyse. At the Province House the mob burns the effigy and a strong wind blows away the ashes, along with the pestilence itself, which, "[i]t was said," abated from that hour. The "it was said" signals Hawthorne's movement away from allegory. He claims that a legend has arisen among the people that a female figure may at times still be seen lurking in the dark corners of a certain chamber of the Province House, its face muffled in an embroidered mantle.

What we have, then, is a confusion of allegory with legend that throws into doubt the moral import of the one and the traditional basis of the other. Allegorically the story turns on the equivalence between the puffed-up sin of pride and the afflictions of the flesh, such as that which Spenser's Red Cross Knight, in book 1, canto 10 of *The Faerie Queene*, must be cured of in the House of Holiness. In Spenser's allegory the cautery of prayer and fasting burns away the Knight's "proud flesh," an actual medical condition that represents for Spenser the sin of pride against which the knight battles. Spenser sustains his allegory even as he includes this medical detail, but Hawthorne, though he tried to emulate the Renaissance poet's allegorical mode, often blurred the correspondences he sought to establish.

In "Lady Eleanore's Mantle" the allegory begins with the contagion of disease and is extended to include the contagion of revolution. Both are attributed to the first and the deadliest of sins. Hawthorne not only succeeds admirably in establishing Lady Eleanore as the personification of pride when she steps on the back of a colonist while extending her hand to the governor, but he also manages to make the physical body of the colonist the locus of her contempt and our attention. We see in the gesture her aristocratic disdain not only for the body of Jervase Helwyse but for the colonial body politic. When those who fete her by their attendance at the governor's ball are said to be the first infected, we conclude that they too are guilty of pride and are thus a source of offense to their fellow colonists. Proud of their associations with those in high places, they are guilty of offering homage to one whom Hawthorne describes as "the proudest of the proud" ("Mantle," 284). As the epidemic spreads to those who were not on the governor's social list, they "raved against the Lady Eleanore, and cried out that her pride and scorn had evoked a fiend" ("Mantle," 284). But the fiend evoked by her pride and scorn is not solely smallpox, it is also the consciousness of social inequities already present in the colony. Ultimately, the hatred of her that flares up among the people provokes the final scene's revolutionary action, which Hawthorne prepares us for by referring to the epidemic as "an unearthly usurper [who] had found his way into the ruler's mansion" ("Mantle," 283).

Although not too much emphasis should be placed on it, a subtext is suggested by the setting in which Helwyse comes face to face with the ruined lady. When he enters her chamber at the invitation of the doctor, Helwyse finds Eleanore "within the silken curtains of a canopied bed," behind which she moans "dolefully of thirst." Unable to recognize his love, he demands to know what "thing" hides behind the curtains: "Heap of diseased mortality, why lurkest thou in my lady's chamber?" On seeing her his madness overtakes him. Hawthorne says, "He shook his finger at the wretched girl, and the chamber echoed, the curtains of the bed were shaken, with his outburst of insane merriment" ("Mantle," 287). Although we know the disease to be smallpox, there is an association of images that points to syphilis; later in the nineteenth century that disease was often invoked by the image of a woman hiding its ravages from her suitors behind her ball mask. The shift from male to female images of syphilis dates to the eighteenth century, however, and Hogarth's engravings that present the female as the representation of the disease may well have been known to Hawthorne.[9] The repeated reference to the bed curtains and the blighted woman's admission of sinfulness to her would-be lover from the deep recesses of that bed at whose limits he stands, cannot fail to suggest a disease of a more sexual nature. Within the overall scheme of the story the suggestion strengthens the pattern of social disorder Hawthorne presents and alludes to yet another overstepping of boundaries that carries with it divine retribution.

Hawthorne is working (as he often does) on two planes: on the moral plane sin brings its deserved consequences, and on the social and political plane the demands of justice exact the same toll. The problem is that however comfortably Hawthorne the Puritan can work on the moral plane, Hawthorne the American, the child of revolution, is made uneasy by his Puritan legacy. For this reason his political radical, Jervase Helwyse (whose surname suggests he is wise in the ways of the devil), is presented as a madman, thus linking the ideas of madness, disease, and criminal behavior, which were also thematically connected in European thought in the eighteenth century. "Wretched lunatic, what do you seek here?" demands the governor when Helwyse storms the Province House in search of Lady Eleanore. "There is nothing here but Death. Back—or you will meet him!" is the governor's warning ("Mantle," 286), and he might as well be warning against rebellion as against smallpox.

The closest thing to rebellion in the story occurs in the final scene: the processional through the streets that culminates with the burning in effigy of Lady Eleanore. But Hawthorne backs away from a blatant identification of this as revolt, for at this point he leaves off his allegory and returns to his earlier suggestion—though he makes it more overtly at this point—that the story is really a legend. Now, a legend is quite different from an allegory and serves a different purpose. Legends derive from myths but are more localized narratives of more recent times. In Europe they have long served to establish traditional regional connections, often through hagiography—stories of Christian saints who are associated with specific localities. When, in the closing lines of his story, Hawthorne speaks of the burning in effigy of the Lady Eleanore and uses the formulaic "it was said that" to introduce the "mysterious connection" between this event and the abatement of the epidemic, he is dealing with the stuff of legend. Yet despite her name, Rochcliffe, which suggests St. Roch, a victim of bubonic plague credited with saving the lives of many in France during the plague years, this repentant sinner can hardly be considered a saint, local or otherwise.[10] The revolutionary act of burning in effigy a member of the British aristocracy is made the subject of a legend probably because Hawthorne could not see it as a moral action suited to allegory. The result, however, is a weakened narrative structure that veers between allegory and legend.

What Hawthorne unintentionally acknowledges by the structural ambiguity of this tale is the void left by the shift of rhetoric away from the earlier strict correspondence between biblical allegory and the political perspective within which the Puritans came to view their mission. The new rhetoric emptied their history of much of its spiritual reference, creating a void that was eventually filled by the political rhetoric of the eighteenth century.

In many of his colonial tales we see Hawthorne struggling toward the symbolic articulation of revolutionary rhetoric, straining to arrive at the figure that will meld, as did the allegorical trope, the disparate strains of Puritanism and rationalism with which he had to work. In "Lady Eleanore's Mantle" he has set himself the task of fusing one subject matter, epidemical disease and contagion—a subject with strong biblical connotations—with another of a purely political nature. In the Puritan biblical allegory one could deal with epidemical disease as the result of sin, thus blending physical and spiritual conditions and making one the consequent of the other. But the task of the American writer was made difficult by the events of a national history that required him to employ the rhetoric of two distinct perspectives, biblical and political. Hawthorne handles his problem by means of the ceremonial action that takes place at the end of the tale. It is a symbolic dramatization of a people acting out of a biblical understanding of epidemic and performing the old ritual of repentance for sin, as well as a reference to the political act of a rebellious people. The ritual of the one lends solemnity to the other so that the political act acquires something of the spirituality of the original biblical interpretation of the Puritan mission. In essence the collective act at the end of "Lady Eleanore's Mantle" is a rite of purification by which the "American" author comes to terms with his divided sensibility.

Hawthorne was unwilling to assert the exact origin of the combination of smallpox and rebellion that he creates in this tale—that is, whether it is pathological (arising from internal disorder) or etiological (remote causation). In part his reluctance stems from the inevitable influence on him of the early nineteenth century's medical discourse, which was still very much caught up in the question of disease causation and leaned heavily in favor of environmentalism. In the context of the story Hawthorne's reluctance to localize the origin of the epidemic is not only a syntactical but a tactical retreat, a rhetorical strategy like those employed by Franklin, whose humor we have long recognized as subversive. "Lady Eleanore's Mantle" merely suggests the connection between the ills of a society and the drastic measures that might be undertaken to remedy them. It avoids a straightforward equation of either aristocracy or rebellion with the epidemic, suggesting instead the kind of relationship already referred to in the *New-England Courant*'s use of the inoculation controversy, that of an opportunistic to a primary infection. Still, the ritual of purification by which the source of primary infection is eradicated from the colony casts the weight of blame on Lady Eleanore.

= Doctors and Revolutionaries =

There is virtually nothing in Hawthorne's tale that speaks, even obliquely, of the actual events of the 1721 epidemic. These he narrated fully in the biography of Cotton Mather written for children and included in the collection *Grandfather's Chair* (1840), employing the straightforward tone and manner he usually adopted for his juvenile readers. But Cotton Mather, the *New-England Courant*, and the inoculation controversy are all lost in the allegory-legend of "Lady Eleanore's Mantle." What we do have are some provocative references to the medical profession. Because of their education and their generally democratic leanings, medical men played active parts in the Revolution and in the newly established Republic; they combined the rationalism of science with politics in ways that appear to have caused Hawthorne some uneasiness. Hawthorne is a nineteenth-century writer, of course, but he betrays here, as elsewhere, a mistrust of that century's expansion of scientific—and pseudo-scientific—theory into the field of social science. In "Lady Eleanore's Mantle" so much of the narrative is given over to the development of an allegory, and the garish embellishments of plot can so distract the reader, that it is easy to overlook the very minor figure in the tale who acts as its voice of reason.

Dr. Clarke is presented as "a physician, and a famous champion of the popular party," a designation Hawthorne makes no further comment on ("Mantle," 275). A first guess might lead one to think that the doctor is part of the group that fostered the *New-England Courant*, but this is not Hawthorne's reference (though the doctor may have been an appreciative reader of the newspaper). In fact, he has combined two Clarkes of the period, one a physician Dr. John Clarke, and the other a politician. The physician, whose surname is sometimes spelled Clark, was a member of a famous family of medical men. In the smallpox epidemic that struck Boston in 1764, an epidemic second only to that of 1721, he administered inoculations, a fact that no doubt caused Hawthorne to associate him with Cotton Mather's earlier advocacy of that practice. The second Clarke is John Clarke, a political enemy of Gov. Shute at the time of the 1721 epidemic. His position as speaker of the State House of Representatives at the time of the outbreak probably would account for Hawthorne's description of his Dr. Clarke as a "champion of the popular party." Certainly within the context of the story his role is far more political than medical.

Since the doctor is said to represent the people in the State House, Hawthorne may be offering in him a sign of their rebellious, democratic spirit. As might be expected from a man of science, Dr. Clarke is the only one who keeps a cool head while the singular events of the tale flow around him. He is also the one who speaks harsh truth, beginning with his first utterance. When Lady Eleanore arrives in Boston a funeral is in progress; the customary peal of welcome for distinguished visitors cannot be rung from the bell of Old South Church, which is sounding the funeral tone. Hence, Hawthorne says, the lady was ushered into the colony by this doleful sound, "as if calamity had come embodied in her beautiful person." The "as if" signals Hawthorne's technique of suggesting alternative interpretations of events. An English officer expresses annoyance at the unhappy coincidence, voicing the opinion that the funeral should have been deferred, and at this point Dr. Clarke enters the story. He begs the officer's pardon for contradicting him and, alluding to the harsh medical fact of decaying flesh, reminds him that "a dead beggar must have precedence of a living queen. King Death confers high privileges" ("Mantle," 276).

The truism in the leveling of all ranks by the dictates of mortality is borne out by the subsequent events of the story, but Dr. Clarke has his own further thoughts on the topic. Told by the officer that the unfortunate youth, Jervase Helwyse, is mad to aspire to the Lady Eleanore, the doctor frowns and says that it may be so, but that he will doubt the justice of Heaven if no "signal humiliation" overtakes the haughty lady. And at this point he describes her in the precise terms that Helwyse will later use: as someone who has sought "to place herself above the sympathies of our common nature, which envelops all human souls." "See, if that nature do not assert its claim over her," he predicts, "in some mode that shall bring her level with the lowest" ("Mantle," 276). Later, when Helwyse offers the lady the communion cup, his words are, "And this shall be a symbol that you have not sought to withdraw yourself from the chain of human sympathies—which whoso would shake off must keep company with fallen angels" ("Mantle," 280).

The strong similarity between these two statements supports the notion that Dr. Clarke and Helwyse are confederates in their opposition to the governor.[11] Invited as a matter of courtesy perhaps (we learn later that the doctor is an infrequent guest at the Province House), we can only imagine that Dr. Clarke attends the ball out of the same sense of protocol. The doctor keeps his distance from the guest of honor, however, observing her, or as Hawthorne puts it, "eyeing her with such keen sagacity that Captain Langford involuntarily gave him credit for the discovery of some deep secret" ("Mantle," 281). It is an instance of that medical gaze to which Foucault has attached great import, and the doctor's observation, from a deliberately maintained distance, is the more crucial here since it creates the impression, in the mind of the captain at least, that the doctor has gained some secret knowledge of the lady. In fact, the officer attempts to "draw forth the physician's hidden knowledge" ("Mantle," 281). Whether Dr. Clarke has gained a knowledge beyond that of the illness apparent to his eye, neither Capt. Langford nor the reader learns directly. But the echo of his and Helwyse's words in the lady's confession of her sin of pride and her scorn of "the sympathies of nature" strongly suggests that it is this sin that has been revealed to his gaze. Once again Hawthorne alludes to the broader sympathies linking individuals in society by focusing attention on the physical body, bringing to the ancient fear of contagion a new political awareness. Lady Eleanore's aristocratic rejection of her connection to the human community has brought forth a violent rejoinder from nature; the ending of the story, however, suggests that there are those who will not be content to wait for nature to redress their wrongs.

In describing the epidemic of 1721 Hawthorne says that "it was distinguished by a peculiar virulence, insomuch that it has left its traces . . . on the history of the country" ("Mantle," 282). Statements such as this cannot fail to suggest the connection he is establishing between the epidemic and the revolutionary spirit, both of which spread through the colony in the course of his narrative. The frequently noted ambiguity of this tale of smallpox qua rebellion in New England, however, is the result of Hawthorne's middle-ground position between the lady and the revolutionaries. Although his sentiments as an American lead him to seek a foreign source for the epidemic, the way in which political rhetoric proves contagious is demonstrated in the nearly identical words used by Dr. Clarke and Helwyse to describe the Lady Eleanore's pride. Both speak of her having withdrawn herself from the chain of humanity. The doctor, fittingly, refers to a commonality of nature; the more emotive Helwyse alludes to the fallen angels as the only company left to those who forsake their human sympathies—and thus neatly places the lady in the ranks of the rebellious. Their frames of reference may be different, but each levels essentially the same charge against the aristocratic lady: her pride severs her connections to the human community and makes her a source of danger to it. Should we doubt which of the two men has initiated the thought, we only need to look at Hawthorne's description of both of them poised at the threshold of the diseased lady's chamber to establish their relationship to each other. Helwyse wants to kneel before the lady, even in her blighted condition, but the doctor, "moved by a deep sense of human weakness," cannot suppress "a smile of caustic humor [that] curled his lip even then." His sense of superiority to Helwyse's display of human weakness is conveyed in his response, "Thus man doth ever to his tyrants" ("Mantle," 286).

Dr. Clarke has been seen by more than one critic of this tale as the moral equivalent of Lady Eleanore, as guilty of a prideful, rebellious spirit as she is of a prideful, aristocratic one (Liebman, 100; Colacurcio, 439). Certainly there is no doubt of his influence over Jervase Helwyse, and it may be that by such narrative devices as the doctor's harsh statements, cold attitude, caustic humor, and distancing of himself physically and emotionally from others, Hawthorne is suggesting that through science we may also sever our connections to the human community. We are not told whether Dr. Clarke takes part in the concluding processional, but one seriously doubts that he would. The last we see of Dr. Clarke is when he opens a door to the lady's infected chamber, signals to Helwyse that he should enter, and bids him "Call her." It is an act of gross irresponsibility on the part of the man of medicine and suggests his true role—a spreader of political contagion. It is not surprising that Hawthorne should assign to a physician the role of purveyor of noxious ideas, since the misuse of science is a familiar narrative theme in Hawthorne; one thinks of "The Birthmark" (1843), "Rappaccini's Daughter" (1844), and of Roger Chillingworth's power over Arthur Dimmesdale in *The Scarlet Letter* (1850). How such power came to be associated with the world of medicine, and why Hawthorne feared its exercise, is inextricably bound up in the history of epidemics and the development in America of a romantic fiction. Although "Lady Eleanore's Mantle" is not among the first rank of Hawthorne's tales, it has a significant place in that history, as did the smallpox epidemic it ambiguously narrates.

3

The American Plague

WHEN HOLLYWOOD GAVE US SCENES OF A YELLOW FEVER epidemic in the 1939 film *Jezebel*, it was mainly to provide the heroine, played by the remarkable Bette Davis, with an opportunity to redeem herself. The movie's setting is 1850s New Orleans, and the love story involves a willful southern belle whose behavior earns her the name of the biblical character who "did evil in the sight of the Lord." In the closing scenes we are presented with a truly grim picture of a city caught in the throes of a dreaded and highly contagious disease. There is only one place for those who fall ill of this disease, the offshore leprosarium. The description offered by the film's heroine of what it will be like for the fever victims, and whoever accompanies them to this lazaretto, is enough to dissuade anyone from the undertaking, but in the end we see Ms. Davis bravely setting out with the stricken man she loves to what seems certain death for them both.

The heroine of *Jezebel* represents the Old South, a representation shown most vividly in a scene where, dressed in a dazzlingly white ball gown, she leads the plantation slave children in a kind of magnanimous sing-along.

Jezebel's rival, the wife of her erstwhile lover, is a northerner. Out of place in the feudal South, she does not understand slavery or duels or the dreaded fever that causes civilized people to shoot those who would flee the city precincts and thus spread the disease. Only a southerner, only a native of New Orleans, can understand, and so Jezebel, the Old South, is redeemed both by her sacrifice and by her cultural heritage. The film, produced the same year as *Gone With the Wind* (and as a consolation to Ms. Davis, who did not win the role of Scarlett O'Hara), is yet another Hollywood paean to the fortitude of southern women who, like the region they represent, are depicted as possessing deep reservoirs of culturally bred strength.

There is no question of the fever scenario being mere movie scripting, for low-lying New Orleans, with its often stagnant waters, was the scene of many a yellow fever epidemic. George Washington Cable's description of the rush to get out of New Orleans in 1853, the year of that city's worst epidemic, is particularly vivid: "Everywhere porters were tossing trunks into wagons, carriages rattling over the stones and whirling out across the broad white levee to the steamboats' sides. Foot-passengers were hurrying along the sidewalk, luggage and children in hand, and out of breath, many a one with the plague already in his pulse."[1]

In *The Grandissimes* (1879) Cable tells the story of a German-American family of father, mother, two daughters, and a son (the siblings all in young adulthood) who migrate south to establish themselves in New Orleans. The year is 1803, and as the family views the marshy wasteland region of the Mississippi River where they have come to settle, "a whirligig of jubilant mosquitoes spin[s] about each head."[2] Within a fortnight all but the son are dead of yellow fever. The father's comment on the day of arrival, that "[t]hese mosquitoes, children, are thought by some to keep the air pure," seems a bit of novelistic artistry on Cable's part until one realizes that even at the time he wrote, the connection between yellow fever and its mosquito vector had not yet been made.

Yellow fever outbreaks are part of this country's history from its first years as a nation and have become a part of its literature as well. So horrifying was the experience of the 1793 epidemic in Philadelphia that survivors seem to have sought catharsis in writing about it. Mathew Carey, a Philadelphia printer, rushed to publish *A Short Account of the Malignant Fever* in November of the fateful year. Carey's account included a gratuitous indictment of the blacks who served as nurses and grave diggers during the epidemic, eliciting a spirited response from two of the city's black ministers. *Narrative of the Proceedings of the Black People, during the Late Awful Calamity* (1794) by Richard Allen and Absalom Jones, both former slaves, is an important part of yellow fever history as well as an important piece of black history. Noah Webster, who early assumed a statesman's vision, wrote essays on the seriousness of the threat the disease posed to the nation's future. Charles Brockden Brown, the country's first serious novelist, used yellow fever as a major theme in two of his works, and Henry Wadsworth Longfellow found plague-ridden Philadelphia a romantic setting for the reunion of Evangeline and Gabriel in his narrative poem *Evangeline* (1849). The demystification of the disease occurred only in the first decade of the twentieth century, so that S. Weir Mitchell (1829–1914), an American physician and popular writer of his time, was medically topical when he included scenes from the 1793 Philadelphia epidemic in *The Red City* (1907).

The medical literature devoted to this disease began in 1793, the year of the worst yellow fever epidemic in America; the medical record of the Philadelphia epidemic of that year is abundant, with every point of view represented. Outstanding in this body of work are the essays and letters of Dr. Benjamin Rush, the greatest American physician of his time. The historian J. H. Powell brought together into one concise telling the many disparate aspects of the 1793 epidemic in *Bring Out Your Dead* (1949), and in his notes Powell refers the reader to all the primary sources on the subject.

So thrilling was the 1930 development of a successful vaccine by the American medical scientist Wilbur A. Sawyer that modern Americans are more familiar with the conquest of yellow fever than with the havoc it wrought in this country for two centuries. The conquest was an especially inspiring story for a nation battling an economic disaster of plaguelike proportions when playwright Sidney Howard made it the subject of a play during the Great Depression. The play's title, a reference to the flag sailing vessels once had been required to display to indicate the presence of the fever aboard, was *Yellow Jack* (1934).

= *Yellow Jack* =

Sidney Howard's play was based on Paul de Kruif's famous 1926 popularization of some outstanding achievements in medical history, *Microbe Hunters*. A chapter in de Kruif's book tells the story of Walter Reed, head of the U.S. Army Yellow Fever Commission sent by the government to Cuba in 1900 because of an epidemic of yellow fever that had killed more American soldiers than had the Spanish in the recently concluded war. Reed and two assistants, Drs. James Carroll and Jesse Lazear, along with the Cuban national Aristides Agramonte, set about a series of experiments on human subjects to test the hypothesis of a Cuban doctor, Carlos Finlay, that yellow fever was spread by mosquitoes. By Christmas Reed was able to report that there was no longer any doubt on the matter, that the essential factor in the infection of a given population is the presence of mosquitoes that have previously bitten humans already infected with yellow fever.[3]

It needed little of the dramatist's skill to turn this thrilling discovery into stage material, but Howard brought to it a theatricality heavily dependent upon staging techniques of light and sound that have since become a staple of theater productions. Drawing on the rampant patriotism at the time of the

Spanish-American War—which had brought the problem of yellow fever to the attention of the U.S. government—the playwright underscores the drama of human volunteers nobly stepping forward to participate in the experiment by filling the theater with the strains of John Philip Sousa's march, "Stars and Stripes Forever."[4] Unfortunately, the conquest of yellow fever is depicted as another victory for Uncle Sam over a foreign enemy rather than an advance in the long struggle of humankind against the tyranny of epidemical disease. But to a people caught in a national depression, the "government to the rescue" theme was no doubt reassuring.

Howard's account of the Cuban expedition against yellow fever makes no reference to the fact that it made possible the building of the Panama Canal, completed in 1914. This long-held political and economic objective of the U.S. government might well have been thwarted indefinitely were it not for the knowledge of the fever gained by the Yellow Fever Commission in Cuba. Nor was yellow fever the sole epidemical threat to the canal's completion: flea-bearing rats caused an outbreak of bubonic plague among the workers (speedily brought under control), and malaria made work on the project all but impossible at times. In sum, the toll in human misery far exceeded that portrayed in Howard's play.

The dream of a canal to link the Atlantic and Pacific oceans at the Isthmus of Panama began with the Spanish conquistadors in 1513. Spain abandoned the idea as too costly (as well as for religious reasons—what God had not done man should not attempt), but it was taken up by the French in the nineteenth century after Spanish influence declined in Central America. Although France had the necessary mechanical and technical skills, evidenced by its successful completion of the Suez Canal, French medical knowledge was insufficient and the attempt was abandoned. The same fate would have attended subsequent efforts by the United States if the team of doctors working in Havana from 1898 to 1902 had not discovered the connection between mosquitoes and malaria and yellow fever. In 1904 one of these doctors, Col. William C. Gorgas, was appointed chief sanitary officer to the Isthmian Commission by President Theodore Roosevelt. Under Gorgas's reorganization of the system of public health in the regions surrounding the future canal, the breeding grounds of mosquitoes were eliminated, screening was introduced, and strict supervision of the sick was undertaken to prevent the spread of yellow fever. Gorgas's campaign eradicated yellow fever by January 1906, a medical conquest of major proportions that made the building of the canal possible.[5]

=   "Fever"   =

The events of the 1793 yellow fever epidemic in Philadelphia serve as the basis of a recent short story. Although John Edgar Wideman's "Fever" (1989) has its own rationale both as fiction and as a "meditation on history" from an African-American point of view, it is dependent on a much earlier account, the little-known record of the 1793 epidemic by the Rt. Rev. Richard Allen and his fellow laborer in the Gospel, Absalom Jones.

Allen was born in Philadelphia in 1760, a slave in the home of a Quaker lawyer. In 1783 he was licensed to preach by the Methodist Society in Delaware, where he was living; he later returned to Philadelphia, still a member of the Methodist Society. As the black membership of the Philadelphia Methodist church increased, largely as a result of Allen's preaching, their number proved threatening to the white congregants, who asked them at one worship service to remove themselves from a prominent position to one less prominent, the gallery, where they would not be seen. At a later service Allen and other African-Americans were pulled from their knees while in prayer and told not to worship there any longer. Allen left and went on to found the African Methodist Episcopal (AME) Church. He died in 1831 but left a record of what he called *The Life Experience and Gospel Labors of the Rt. Rev. Richard Allen*, to which is appended the *Narrative of the Proceedings of the Black People . . .* , a straightforward account of the part the two authors and other blacks had played during the Philadelphia epidemic.

Wideman dedicates his story to Mathew Carey, who fled Philadelphia in its hour of need and on his return published a libelous account of black nurses and undertakers, those pressed into service and volunteers alike. Carey's accusation of their profiteering during the epidemic injured, as Allen wrote, "all people of my race and especially those without whose unselfish, courageous labours the city could not have survived the late calamity."[6]

Below the dedication to Carey, Wideman has added a 1777 quotation from Robert Morris, who compares Philadelphia (soon to become the capital of the new nation) in its centrality of industry and commerce to the function of the heart in the human body. In drawing on the age-old analogy between the body and the body politic, Wideman immediately points to the literary conventions that associate epidemic disease with societal wrongdoing and thus signals the primary objective of his narrative. This objective is occasionally impeded by the multiple applications of his theme across a variety of historical periods. Before the story has ended we are in Philadelphia some 200 years later, after the 1985 police bombing of the headquarters of a radical inner-city commune that called itself MOVE, resulting in the deaths of women and children who were members of the commune.

Despite the overextension, the story makes effective use of quotations from *Narrative of the Proceedings . . .* and of multiple narrative voices, which demand of the reader the kind of attention Allen and Jones might have wished from the white citizens of their city in 1794. Among the narrative voices, for example, is that of a Jew who excoriates the fictional Allen, as the latter attends his dying, for being a slave to his sense of "duty and obligation" ("Fever," 155). Wideman provides definitions of yellow fever and of dengue and discusses the eighteenth century's confusion of these two diseases; he also mentions the government's attempt to associate yellow fever with the slave insurrection in Santo Domingo. Wideman's principal analogy, however, is drawn from the more modern conclusion that yellow fever was imported into this country from Africa as a by-product of the slave trade. Thus he has Allen speak of yellow fever as a parallel to that other "fever," the one that "grows in the secret places of our hearts, planted there when one of us decided to sell one of us to another" ("Fever," 133).

The "us," of course, extends the metaphor to all humankind, making the evil of slavery a sin against humanity; sin, like the yellow fever, is peculiar to no one race. Another narrative device that works to establish universality appears to derive from Foucault's use of quotations from medical literature in *Birth of the Clinic*—notably, that work's description of the membranous tissue covering the brain of a patient dead of meningitis (*Foucault* ix). "When you open the dead, black or white, you find: the dura mater covering the brain is white and fibrous in appearance," Wideman begins one section of his narrative, the remainder of which is an autopsy report on a yellow fever victim, including the weight of each vital organ and the aspect of every interior part of the body from the viewpoint of the dissector. Here, indeed, is the medical gaze of which Foucault speaks, and linked quite overtly to the authorial voice. It is a viewpoint that, as shall be seen, has its origins in literature contemporary with the yellow fever epidemics of the 1790s.

Wideman's story is both an excellent evocation of the Allen and Jones narrative and a purposeful expansion of its self-imposed limitations. Whereas the black ministers had sought to argue their case in a restrained account, providing factual evidence of their work and figures for monies received for services rendered the sick and the dead, Wideman goes behind this factual facade to explore the feelings of the two men. The original narrative conveys a deep sense of injured pride and an almost irreparable hurt at the charges of Mathew Carey. Wideman expands upon these emotions to consider the sacrifice Allen made in leaving his own family and his own people to minister to whites suffering in the worst of conditions, all of whom profited in some way from a society that allowed slavery.

At the deepest level Wideman's story reveals an awareness of the uses to which a plague narrative can be put—advancing political ends, driving home a moral, or serving as a "meditation on history," as he says. "Fever" is the latest fictional attempt to define the essence of the yellow fever experience in eighteenth-century America, but the effort began long ago, contemporaneously with the worst outbreaks of the disease and with the inception of romantic fiction in America.

= Friendship in a Time of Plague =

"Why do you so much delight in Mystery? Is it the disease of Will? or of Habit? . . . The man of Truth, Charles! the pupil of Reason, has no mysteries."[7] The object of this stern admonition was Charles Brockden Brown, America's first author of romantic fiction; his admonisher was Dr. Elihu Hubbard Smith, a friend who had great plans for Brown—he was to be the creator of an American literature of reason. The year was 1796, the new Republic had need of a man of letters, and Dr. Smith was perceptive enough to see Brown's potential, both as a writer and as an advocate of republican causes. By using his influence with fellow New Englanders, Smith hoped to place his friend's writings in such staunchly Federalist (hence conservative) newspapers as Joseph Dennie's *The Farmer's Weekly Museum*. Not only was Smith seeking an audience for Brown among the more educated in the nation, he was hoping as well to spread among them the liberal doctrines of republican rationalism. From this relationship between the doctor and the writer there arose a dialogical literature rooted in the conflict between the rationalist discourse of the eighteenth century and a nascent romanticism. Before it was ended by a personal tragedy involving yellow fever, their relationship had affected the carryover into American fiction of the allegorical impulse already present in American thought and had raised serious questions about the power bases in American society.

Elihu Hubbard Smith was a native of Litchfield, Connecticut. He had been part of the second tier of "Hartford Wits," who were all well educated (Yale College), from good families, and of Federalist persuasion. Their efforts on behalf of the ratification of the Constitution led them into a defense of what they considered marks of the true American: a reverence for the order established by that document, and an abhorrence of anything that would further disturb the New England way of life. This passion for order—which also permeated Smith's private life—led to an equal passion for knowledge, categorized and systematized knowledge designed to dispel the riddles of human experience. To Smith's way of thinking, the mysteries of the universe would always yield to a rational understanding.

Eventually Smith's rationalism took the form of democratic republicanism, a political stance to which he was driven by the influence of Calvinism on New England Federalism. After losing all faith in Christianity while at Yale (a loss his parents tried, unsuccessfully, to rectify by enrolling him in Timothy Dwight's Greenfield Hill School), Smith moved steadily in the direction of faith in reason and in science. It was while he was attending lectures given at Pennsylvania Hospital by Dr. Benjamin Rush that Smith met Charles Brockden Brown.

Brown was a native of Philadelphia; of Quaker background (though a nonbeliever), he had been educated in the law but chose not to practice it. Brown wanted to be a writer. His initial plans for an epic poem had not materialized, but he quickly fell in with Smith's plans for the production of literary pieces to be submitted to leading journals and newspapers. The two young men were radically different in temperament, however. While Smith waited impatiently in New York City, where he had set up medical practice, for literary examples of what he referred to—with emphasis—as "*the truth*," Brown wrote him letters filled with mysterious references to events and people of his imagining. The doctor's response was to equate (as in the admonition that opens this chapter) such romantic productions with disease.

For men such as Elihu Smith and his mentor Dr. Rush, the mysteries surrounding disease were susceptible to illumination by the scientific mind; it was merely a matter of time before all would be known and understood. For Charles Brockden Brown, no such certainty existed; rather, all was mystery and shadow, including his chosen occupation as a writer. There was no "American" writer after whom he could pattern himself, and there was no American society about which, in emulation of British writers, he might write. America as a literary subject, other than as a newly created political entity, did not properly exist. With little of substance to inspire him, it is not surprising that Brown embraced shadow.

Yet it is a disservice to his talent, and to the critical abilities of scholars who have universally hailed him, not to acknowledge the great extent to which Brown's romances reflect the most philosophically and politically advanced ideas of his time. Brown was an urbanite who lived most of his life in Philadelphia, the nation's capital, and for a time with Smith in New York. Fluent in French, he read and supported French revolutionary thought and fashioned literary characters out of intellectual arguments; many of his romances are enacted dialogue between opposing philosophies—virtual allegories, in fact, of the ongoing dialogue in which he and Smith engaged. Despite the intellectual content of these fictions, however, they are highly romantic. What brings them to our attention anew, to be reexamined in light of recent theorizing, is the fact that they are romances whose themes are madness, death, epidemical disease, sex, and—always—power.

The romances came close together—four between 1798 and 1800, followed a few years later by two sentimental novels of little value or importance. The first of the four, *Wieland* (1798), is a depiction of madness as an inherited tendency that finds its outlet in the sacrificial slaughter of a family. The second, *Ormond* (1799), pits a rational heroine against an irrational, power-driven member of a secret society who threatens her virtue and her life, causing her to commit murder in self-defense. The third, *Arthur Mervyn* (1799–1800), is a historical romance based, like Wideman's "Fever," on the Philadelphia yellow fever epidemic of 1793. The fourth, *Edgar Huntly* (1799), combines murder, madness, and detection with a depiction of natural landscape as a psychological correlative of all three.

Embedded in each of the romances is the ideological contest that developed between Smith and Brown. Two of them feature the yellow fever epidemics of the 1790s. Unlike Daniel Defoe, whose classic work on the 1665 Great Plague of London, *A Journal of the Plague Year*, is not the contemporary account it appears to be (Defoe was only five years old at the time of the bubonic plague), Brown lived through and experienced firsthand the decade of the American plague, and for some time the subject dominated his thinking. I will argue here that the psychological landscape in *Edgar Huntly* reflects Brown's fear of yellow fever and his lack of faith in the ability of science to "know," with certainty, its cause.

A crucial difference between Smith and Brown reveals itself in the spontaneity with which Brown's heroes and heroines make moral choices after having considered opposing points of view; such spontaneity and autonomy were denied by Smith's view of man as "an improving animal" (the belief also held by Benjamin Franklin and Joseph Priestley) capable of being habituated to moral behavior. This theory of perfectibility informs the character of the villainous Ormond, in Brown's romance of that title, who claims to have attained a level of human capability far beyond the norm. Though he offers no evidence of a concomitant moral improvement, Ormond insists he has so advanced his faculties that it is possible for him to perceive the actions of others without their awareness. Brown subtitled his romance, *The Secret Witness*; it is the first indication of his fear of the rationalist, scientific gaze.

Brown might be thought to have been merely caught up in a sort of love-hate relationship with a rather formidable mentor were it not for the deadly serious turn of events that cast a new light not only on his friendship with Smith but on everything in his social environment. The events were those associated with the series of yellow fever epidemics that became the fulcrum on which turned all social and political life in the nation. So all-encompassing were the effects of the epidemics that they assumed proportions unlike those of any other event in the history of the young Republic.

= A Climate of Fear =

According to the most reliable evidence, yellow fever entered the New England colonies in 1693, brought into Boston Harbor, it is believed, by British trading ships from Barbados. In the eighteenth century there were major outbreaks in Charleston, New York, and Philadelphia. These occurrences reached a peak in 1745, diminished in frequency until about 1760, and then disappeared until 1793. The sudden reappearance of the disease after some 30 years, and its unpropitious timing, so soon after the establishment of the Republic, was a source of great consternation to citizens of the new nation. When the years 1791, 1793, 1794, 1795, 1797, and 1798 all saw epidemics of yellow fever in cities ranging as far apart as New Haven, Connecticut, and

Charleston, South Carolina, the hopes and bright visions of America as "a fairer Pisgah," as Philip Freneau and Hugh Henry Brackenridge named it in their 1786 poem, "The Rising Glory of America," began to fade.[8] Worst of all, from the perspective of the new citizenry, Europeans had begun referring to the disease as "the American plague."

What made yellow fever especially terrifying was that, unlike smallpox, it was not known in Europe. An infectious, viral disease found in subtropical and tropical areas, it is transmitted by female mosquitoes of the genus *Aëdes aegypti*. The onset of the fever is sudden, with accompanying headache, nausea, and nosebleeds. Later the eyes take on a yellow cast, which gives the fever its name. With this comes great straining of the stomach, which produces hemorrhaging and a subsequent black vomit caused by accumulations of stale blood. The lymph nodes, especially under the arms and in the groin, often swell to the point of bursting, producing the buboes originally named for their appearance in bubonic fever.

The cause of this fever was a mystery that aroused in Americans the worst fears of nature as a threat to their survival. The origins of this fear lay in the anti-nature image of America created by a Europe that found the overwhelming abundance of wild, untamed nature in the New World distasteful. The "true relations" penned by Renaissance travelers, in which were described all manner of natural wonders, both beautiful and terrifying, to be found in America, were transmuted into legends that circulated in the villages of European nations. New England Puritanism furthered the image, but later the institution of a self-proclaimed Republic of virtue and the growth of a self-conscious national pride gave rise to deliberate attempts to blend the double view of nature in America, as in Timothy Dwight's *The Conquest of Canaan* (1785) and Joel Barlow's *The Vision of Columbus* (1787).

America's natural environment was a matter of no small importance to the new Republic, especially given the widespread belief in Montesquieu's claim, articulated in his *L'Espirit des lois* (1748), that a nation's climate is the deciding factor in its prosperity. This environmentalist theory gradually widened to include, as part of its "climate," a society's institutions. Just one year after the colonies declared their independence, and when interest in America was at a peak, the English historian William Robertson published his *History of America* (1777), which repeated the earlier findings of such naturalists as Buffon, Kalm, Raynal, and De Pauw.[9] Though only the Swedish botanist Pehr Kalm had visited the New World, each of these authors had written of it with varying degrees of negativity. The most sensational was Corneille De Pauw's two-volume work, which never deviated from its thesis, offered on the first page: *"C'est sans doute, un spectacle grand et terrible de voir une moitié de ce globe, tellement disgraciée par la nature, que tout y étoit ou dégénéré, ou monstrueux"* (*Recherches*, I, 1 [my translation]; "Without a doubt, it is a grand and terrible spectacle to behold half of the globe so disgraced by nature, that everything in it tends toward degeneracy or monstrosity"). Pronouncements such as this one haunted Americans, and the yellow fever epidemics appeared to give them credence.

Although numerous modern studies offer ample information on the horrors and the wide-ranging impact of these epidemics, the present purpose is better served by C. F. Volney's *A View of the Soil and Climate of the United States of America*, published in Philadelphia in 1804. The translator of this edition was Charles Brockden Brown, whose footnotes provide a running refutation of Volney's discussion of the disease. Brown had known Volney while the Frenchman was in America. A refugee of the revolutionary dictatorship of Danton and Robespierre, he arrived in Philadelphia in the fall of 1795. Volney traveled extensively throughout the United States before writing his book and acknowledged a great debt to Dr. Samuel Latham Mitchill of New York for his work on geology and climate in the States. Mitchill was Elihu Hubbard Smith's coeditor in the publication of the nation's first medical journal, *The Medical Repository*, and a friend to Brown. Despite these native influences, Volney's account of America's climate is written in the same vein as those of his earlier compatriots.

Brown's editorial comments contradict almost all of Volney's findings, but his ire becomes most evident in chapter 10, "Of the reigning Diseases in the United States," where the Frenchman reviews the two medical theories of yellow fever formulated in the States during the epidemic years. The two theories were rooted in the conflicting views of contagion represented by the sixteenth-century Italian physician Girolamo Fracastoro, who believed such diseases were communicated through direct contact with sick individuals or their clothing, and by the seventeenth-century English physician Thomas Sydenham, who advocated the "miasmic theory" that in certain places noxious elements rose from the earth to taint the air. In the eighteenth-century debate on the cause of yellow fever, these were known as the contagionist and the environmentalist views. By the first theory, yellow fever was an infectious, contagious disease imported from an outside source, probably the West Indies. The second theory claimed the fever was of local origin, not inherent in the nature of America but the result of miasmic vapors rising from the preponderance of filth that daily accumulated in the cities of the eastern seaboard. Since these cities were not only sites of the fever's repeated outbreak but also the vital shipping ports of the nation, both the importationist and local-origin theories had to be considered with a view to their effects on the nation's economy. Needless to say, the local-origin theory was far from acceptable to the Federalist government.

Belief in quarantine is as old as the awareness of contagious disease. (The word originates in the Italian *quarantina*, which refers to the 40 days ships believed to be carrying disease were kept out of Italian ports.) Damaging though the practice of quarantine would have been to the shipping interests of the nation, it was viewed by the importationists as a temporary measure that would have created no overall or lasting damage to the mercantile businesses.

General acceptance of the idea that yellow fever originated in American cities, however, would cause foreign ships to avoid those cities and make American ships unwelcome in foreign ports. Further, the anticontagionists, with their talk of miasmic influences in the air, sounded to many like spiritualists rather than men of science, and their admonitions about greater cleanliness met with resistance and open hostility from a people oblivious to the existence of microbes. One instance of the shortsightedness that prevailed in the city of Philadelphia was the reluctance by religious societies to accept the installation of public bathhouses, because they believed them to be "unfriendly to morals" (Shryock, 91).

The controversy took on wider implications as the death toll rose in the 1790s, until eventually the origin of yellow fever had become a political, religious, and moral issue as well as a medical problem. In 1793 the death count by the time of the first frost, which always ended the sieges, was at least 5,000, a figure that represented roughly 10 percent of the city's population. When questions were raised as to why the fever had returned with such virulence, it was not long before fingers were pointed at the 2,000 refugees from Santo Domingo who—fleeing slave revolts and yellow fever in their native island—had arrived in Philadelphia that summer. All such facts and coincidences fed the controversy generated by the competing explanations for the epidemic, internal versus external, the contagionist versus the environmentalist, the importationist view versus the local-origin theory.

In his account Volney indicates his belief in the local-origin theory and his doubt that the fever was in all cases contagious. Charles Brockden Brown takes a very negative attitude, however, toward Volney's review of the controversy, denigrating the French author's remarks on both points. Moreover, in one editorial note he questions both the importationist and the local-origin arguments by asking: "Why, exclaims one, did not the equal or greater filth and impurity of our towns generate the fever before 1790? and why, may another exclaim, did not our intercourse with the West Indies import that disease sooner? an intercourse more incautious and unguarded than at present."[10] A few pages later he adds a personal attack on Volney as one of those "violent controversialists [who] have not minds large enough to see the real complexity and obscurity of this question, or to admit the possibility of opposite opinions being adopted or defended with disinterested motives" (*View*, 252n). Ultimately Brown dismisses both hypotheses, but with a particularly telling blow aimed at the scientific rationalists who constituted the local-origin coterie: "The rage for explaining every thing, and the dogmatic spirit that imagines the causes of every thing within our reach, is as prevalent now as in the darkest ages of the world" (*View*, 249n).

Obviously, by 1803 Brown no longer shared the belief of most of his countrymen in history as a steady progress toward a brighter future but viewed it instead as a cyclical process of periodic returns to a darker age.

Behind this response lay a bitter personal experience that had ultimately confirmed his adherence to romance and mystery rather than to the rational beliefs of his medical friend Elihu Smith.

Although the epidemic of 1793 became the premise of his novel *Arthur Mervyn, or, Memoirs of the Year 1793*, Brown was not actually in Philadelphia during that worst of the yellow fever epidemics. He prudently left the city, as did thousands of others, and stayed with Elihu Smith at the home of Smith's parents in Litchfield, Connecticut. Later, in 1795, during the epidemic in New York of which he wrote in *Ormond*, he was in Perth Amboy, New Jersey, visiting with the dramatist William Dunlap. In August 1798 Elihu Smith was correcting proofs of *Wieland*, Brown's first romance, and reading a manuscript copy of "Sky-Walk," a romance Brown had finished late in the preceding year. This latter work was being printed in Philadelphia when the epidemic in that city brought death to the publisher and destruction to the printed portion of the book. At the same time that his work was becoming a casualty of the epidemic in Philadelphia, Brown and two friends, Elihu Smith and William Johnson, with whom he was spending the summer, came under the same baneful shadow in New York.

Never one to withhold judgment on any subject, Smith had formed firm opinions on every aspect of the yellow fever controversy, an issue that had become bound up with another that also caused major division between Americans—the war between France and England. The official position of the U.S. government was one of neutrality, but that did little to stop either the Federalists from continuing their attempts to involve the country in England's behalf, or the Republicans from attempting the same for France. Every local and national issue became a reflection of the international struggle in which America supposedly had no part, and yellow fever, a topic on every tongue, played right into the ideologies of both camps.

The yellow fever epidemics were injected into the political fray because the medical profession, which by and large advocated the theory of local origin, was dominated by Republicans. The importation theory, by contrast, coincided nicely with the Federalist belief that France was in the business of spreading revolution like a plague. With an open declaration of war out of the question, the Federalists settled for amendments to the Naturalization Act and, later, passage of the Alien Act and the Alien Enemies Act. These legislative measures, all enacted in 1798, were designed to draw a political *cordon sanitaire* around the nation. With the passage of the Sedition Act in July of that year, the panic reaction was extended to include citizens of the United States by providing for the imprisonment of anyone, citizen or alien, who attempted to foment insurrection or who wrote, published, or uttered any false or malicious statements against the president, Congress, or the U.S. government.[11] The importationist political coterie had won, and what some saw as the equivalent here of France's Reign of Terror began.

═ The Spread of Revolutionary Fever ═

Pestilence
Written During the Prevalence of a Yellow Fever

Hot, dry winds forever blowing,
Dead men to the grave-yards going:
        Constant hearses,
        Funeral verses;
Oh, what plagues—there is no knowing!
Priests retreating from their pulpits!—
Some in hot, and some in cold fits
        In bad temper,
        Off they scamper,
Leaving us—unhappy culprits!
Doctors raving and disputing,
Death's pale army still recruiting—
        What a pother
        One with t'other!
Some a-writing, some a-shooting,
Nature's poisons here collected,
Water, earth, and air infected—
        O, what pity,
        Such a City,
Was in such a place erected! (Pattee, 110)

So wrote the poet Philip Freneau in Philadelphia in 1793, the same Freneau who in 1786 had written, with Henry Brackenridge, "The Rising Glory of America." As editor of the *National Gazette,* published in Philadelphia, Freneau gave himself over entirely to the cause of revolutionary France, a cause that became increasingly unpopular as affairs there—and in Philadelphia—worsened. Though in the poem he attempts to make light of the situation, he manages to touch on most of the major issues involved in the yellow fever controversy. Especially pointed is his reference to the disputing doctors engaged in their own warfare while death recruits ever more victims. (Freneau further vented his contempt for the medical profession in "On Dr. Sangrado's Flight," a poem castigating one of the doctors who fled Philadelphia in 1793.) In "Pestilence" the poet—predictably—comes down on the Republican side of the controversy and places the blame for the epidemic on the polluted city, thus ranging himself with those environmentalists who proclaimed the fever to be of local origin.

Dr. Elihu Smith also was wholeheartedly in the camp of the local-origin theorists, just as he wholeheartedly favored the Republican supporters of France. Urging a clean environment seemed to him in no way detrimental to America's economic interests since he shared with Benjamin Rush and Benjamin Franklin such Republican notions as the belief that public and private interests in a democracy were identical. His personal involvement in the treatment of those stricken by the fever, by which he hoped to increase his reputation and his practice, was entirely in line with this philosophy.

In his total involvement with the patient and the disease, Smith had as his American model the intrepid Dr. Benjamin Rush, who had abandoned the apolitical, liberal stance of the eighteenth-century gentleman maintained by his colleagues in the Philadelphia College of Physicians in favor of a fervid republicanism. In the fall of 1793, after the epidemic had waned, the college issued an official resolution declaring that yellow fever had never been known to originate in Philadelphia or in any other part of the United States but had in all instances been imported. Rush immediately resigned from its ranks. The college, in turn, censured him for his unorthodox behavior in personally attending, with the aid of nonmedical personnel whom he instructed, victims of the epidemic. Rush further angered the college by persisting in his belief that fever required a reduction of bodily fluids. Throughout his years of practice he wielded the bleeding knife with great abandon and purged his patients repeatedly. This treatment, which came to be known as "the Republican cure," no doubt killed as many as did the fever; nevertheless, Rush was able to gather about him a group of young doctors who eagerly accepted his theory of a local origin for yellow fever.

The search for the mysterious factor to which yellow fever could be linked led the purveyors of the local-origin theory into many a blind alley. Rush thought at one point that it might be the coffee beans left to rot on the Philadelphia docks; Mitchill believed New Yorkers had poisoned their city by using as landfill all manner of garbage and offal. Smith, writing to his fellow physicians in *The Medical Repository*, concluded that the source of the Plague of Athens, described by the historian Thucydides, was local and warned that if such a thing could occur in Athens, the same local causes could "generate a Yellow Fever in Philadelphia—and New York."[12] This was a telling point, for the glories of ancient Rome and Greece were models for the early Republic. Smith knew his Thucydides, as did his fellow doctors. He knew too that most of them shared his rationalist principles, and that they would recall how the historian attributed to the plague the beginnings of a state of lawlessness in Greece, largely because the deaths of good and bad alike eroded faith in the gods. Rationalist or no, Smith was a man who valued public order, and there was nothing that so imperiled it as an epidemic. It was not faith in the gods that was at stake in Philadelphia, the seat of national government, but faith in the government to perform in the best interests of the people. The capital would soon be moved to the new city on the Potomac River, but in the interim, what could be expected of a government that ceased to function at the first signs of epidemic, of public officials who fled and left the people to their own devices? The epidemic of 1793 spawned a host of political and social problems that may have begun with Dr. Rush and his Republican attitudes but soon extended into almost every area of public life.

To begin with, the nonmedical and emergency personnel, including burial teams, who came to the fore during the yellow fever epidemics were mostly blacks. They were solicited for their services, as we know from Richard Allen's narrative, not only because they performed most menial tasks in the society but because it was generally believed they were immune to the disease. There were two bases for this belief: the observation that blacks from the West Indies seemed not to contract yellow fever, and confusion between dengue, a tropical disease also transmitted by the mosquito, and yellow fever. Modern medicine has explained this seeming immunity: we now recognize that the blood cell mutation termed sickle-cell anemia is a racial genetic disorder resulting from an adaptation to the *Aëdes aegypti* mosquito, which transmits both yellow fever and dengue (McNeill, 47).

Emergency personnel also included other men and women of the lower classes, many of them French or Irish immigrants whose national origins led them to be associated in the minds of Federalists with another feared disease, the contagious revolutionary fever, referred to by the Federalists as "the *morbus Gallicus*," an allusion to the Jacobin ascendancy in France in the same year as the Philadelphia epidemic. Although most of these emergency workers were financially unable to leave the cities during times of epidemic, many stayed because they shared the Republican belief in the environmental cause of the disease and therefore discounted the idea of contagion. Because the fate of many of those who died of the fever was determined by either their poverty or their political belief, yellow fever became the first political issue to divide American citizens along social and economic lines. Not even the churches saw fit to offer assistance; indeed, one published discussion, *A Theological Dissertation on the Propriety of Removing from the Seat of the Pestilence; Presented to the Perusal of the Serious Inhabitants of Philadelphia and New-York*, argued that no one was bound to stay and help the sick and poor and reminded those who could not leave the cities that "those who remove to other places suffer too, loss of comfort and substance," so the evacuees were not truly fleeing God's judgment.[13] The author, a minister of the Gospel, even quotes from Cotton Mather's *Magnalia Christi Americana* (1702) to establish that the Puritan divine excused ministers from entering infected sickrooms.

When the 1793 epidemic subsided, those individuals who had set up a provisional government, known simply as the Committee, to secure public services in the absence of the fleeing members of city, state, and federal government, were criticized by the returning Federalists as "upstarts" seeking political advantage. Great efforts were made to undermine the performance record during the emergency of any who later became candidates for public office. One such "upstart" Republican, Israel Israel, who gave unstintingly of his time and labor during the worst weeks of the epidemic, used his "plague record" as a platform in the fall elections. The overwhelming support he received from grateful citizens of his district was overturned by the returning Federalists, who demanded that a new date be set for the voting because of the plague-related absence of many at election time. Israel never did gain elected office, but he remained a thorn in the Federalist side for years to come.[14] The importance of Israel and others who served on the Committee was not to be measured by their future accomplishments, however, but by the fact that in the absence of those officials entrusted with governance, there had emerged—from the general populace—new leadership.

The Federalists drew their strongest support from among the wealthy, who were able to leave the city and escape the epidemic. Money, or the lack of it, so often determined who lived and who died in the epidemics of the 1790s that the economic stratification of the population could hardly be ignored. Those who maintained summer homes outside the city went to them at the first hint of the fever. Those condemned to remain in the city without food supplies or adequate medical services died by the thousands. Charles Brockden Brown refers directly to these social differences. In *Ormond* one of the characters claims, "For the rich, the whole world is a safe asylum; but for us, indigent and wretched, what fate is reserved but to stay and perish?"[15] In *Arthur Mervyn* the common graves of the victims of the fever, "the pits opened alike for the rich and the poor, the known and the unknown," suggest that the only true equality in the new society was the democracy of death.[16] As these two quotations suggest, the subject of yellow fever is treated as the problem of the poor in *Ormond*, and in *Arthur Mervyn* as the problem of the general population. In the former it shapes but a portion of the plot and is only one of many vicissitudes Brown's heroine must overcome in her struggle against adversity. But in *Arthur Mervyn* the epidemic is all-pervasive, supplying the central theme upon which turns the entire narrative.

= *Arthur Mervyn, or,* = Memoirs of the Year 1793

Arthur Mervyn is in two parts; the first begins with the narration of a Dr. Stevens, who relates that, while the city of Philadelphia was beset by an epidemic, he befriended a young man, Arthur Mervyn, whom he found in the street outside his home, obviously ill of a pestilential fever. When Arthur recovers as a result of the doctor's care, he begins his narrative: his childhood (he is but 18) as a country boy, his arrival in the city, and his subsequent employment by a wealthy man who involved the youth in his criminal activities as a counterfeiter. After breaking free of his employer, Arthur had made his way back to his country home but returned to the city at the outbreak of yellow fever to search for the brother of a young woman for whom he has formed a deep affection.

At his reentry into Philadelphia, Arthur sees mankind at its worst, both those who are suffering and those who are inflicting it on others. As he makes his way through the streets of the nearly deserted city noxious odors rise, and he claims "not so much to smell as to taste the element that now encompassed me. . . . Some fatal influence appeared to seize upon my vitals; and the work of corrosion and decomposition to be busily begun" (*Mervyn*, 144). The overwhelming corrosive influence, so physically palpable on his return to the city, has been adumbrated in his initial entry, when he was similarly overwhelmed by the power of wealth to corrode his moral being. For Arthur's participation in his former employer's activities had not been entirely innocent. Though he had made attempts to undo the wrong to which he had been party, the state of his infected body at the outset of the story is the reflection of an earlier moral corruption.

When Arthur ventures into the city at the height of the epidemic, he learns the extent to which the disease of self-interest—the cause of his moral decline—contributes to the epidemical disease and its horrors. He sees the poor who have been left to fend for themselves in the worst of conditions; he sees the burning flesh of those who have not even a cup of water to ease their fever; he sees the dying at the Bush Hill lazaretto whom Brown, following Mathew Carey's account, places at the mercy of callous attendants whose sole reason for being there is the payment offered for their services. Arthur sees that women, children, the elderly, and the poor, all the weakest of society's members, are the prime targets of this double tyranny of disease and selfishness. From a benevolent Quaker who has offered his help to those in need Arthur learns that the origin of the fever can be imputed "not to infected substances imported from the east or west, but to a morbid constitution of the atmosphere, owing wholly, or in part to filthy streets, airless habitations and squalid persons" (*Mervyn*, 161). By thus openly endorsing the theory of local origin Brown includes the Federalist government in his indictment of the self-interest that ruled the nation.

More practically, by removing the source of the epidemic from the realm of the mysterious—and the theurgical—to the realm of the natural, Brown resituates it within the sphere of human activity, wherein lies the means of its eradication. This activity forms the action of part 2 of *Arthur Mervyn*, in which the recovered Arthur sets about the business of cleaning up the city's moral atmosphere. His adventures are too numerous and episodic to recount in detail; suffice to say that Arthur brings light and cleanliness to every dark corner of a society that claims to be virtuous, but whose virtue is as counterfeit as the bills Arthur had once helped circulate.

As a literary work, *Arthur Mervyn* has held up under the test of scholarly criticism; most critics praise Brown for the blend of realism and romance that the work achieves. In the nineteenth century, however, it was considered inferior to *Wieland* (his first romance), which deals with madness as an inherited trait. But it was as "the author of Arthur Mervyn" that in "The Hall of Fantasy" (1846) Nathaniel Hawthorne singled Brown out for a place in his imaginary writers' hall of fame, and with good reason. Few readers would have been more appreciative than Hawthorne of Brown's success in devising a metaphoric image capable of bearing the weight of the multiple associations his society had brought to yellow fever.

Arthur Mervyn is already infected when Brown introduces him. To be infected, as in the Latin *infectio*, means to be stained, tainted, spoiled, or polluted. It is certainly an inauspicious beginning for the first representative hero in American fiction, in what might be called an Arthurian tale set in the new Republic of virtue. Further, this Arthur is stained and polluted by his country's prevailing fever, the epidemical yellow fever, which Brown transforms into a morally corrosive fever of self-interest. It is an apt metaphor, for all sides in the fever controversy sought to advance a partisan interest. Brown defuses the controversy—first, by refusing to consider any explanation for the presence of yellow fever other than the local-origin theory, and second, by dissolving all the medical, political, and religious differences into the one triumphant image of a plague-ridden American who survives.

Arthur's survival is crucial, and not only because survival is a theme repeated often in American literature after Brown. It is important in the context of Brown's own time and experience and owes much to his early acceptance of the ideas of Elihu Smith. In *Arthur Mervyn* the doctor who discovers Arthur in the street and immediately recognizes from his symptoms that his disease is "pestilential" saves Arthur's life by taking him into his own home and treating him. Diagnosis is made on the basis of observation, just as Arthur later diagnoses the illness of his society by firsthand observation of its victims: he sees the sick, the poor, the weak. And when Arthur has recovered from yellow fever, his lengthy narrative of his experiences on coming to the city is the equivalent of a patient's narration of his illness (in this case a moral as well as physical illness) to a doctor. In Foucault's terms (regarding the localizing change that occurred in the late eighteenth century in the question with which the medical interview began), Arthur's answer to the query "Where do you hurt?" is, in effect, "in the city of Philadelphia, capital of the United States of America." From that point Brown is able to promote the local-origin theory *and* fulfill the role of moralist by drawing the analogy between yellow fever and self-interest. The concerns of both doctor and writer are thus served.

= Dr. Elihu Hubbard Smith =

The influence of Elihu Hubbard Smith and his adherence to the Republican local-origin theory of yellow fever can be felt throughout *Arthur Mervyn*. In fact, had he lived, Smith might have exerted, through the amazing number of contacts he maintained with people in every phase of public life in early America, the same kind of influence in many directions. Highly intelligent, full of an energy belied by his physical stature and general state of health, he was idealistic about every phase of his nation's future. Though allowed to use the title "Doctor," Smith was not a physician, as was Dr. Benjamin Rush. His background included work in his father's apothecary shop in Litchfield, but his medical education was limited to a series of lectures given by Rush. Once settled in his New York City practice, however, he devoted himself assiduously to his profession and read extensively in the field. In particular he gave himself over to the study of yellow fever, its manifestations, its similarities to other fevers present and past, and, above all, its probable cause. In addition to his medical interests, he served as secretary for the Manumission Society, edited a volume of American poems—the first in the nation— wrote one play, which was performed once, wrote volumes of letters, kept a diary that is amazing for its detailed information, regularly attended a round of club meetings, and managed to steady Charles Brockden Brown's fits of moodiness while encouraging his friend's writing. Smith even managed to combine his love of literature with his medical interests by composing a series of sonnets in 1797 on subjects pertaining to his environmentalist beliefs. Rather than the usual love lyrics, his sonnets are on the topics of exercise, cold bathing, exercise, proper dress, and cleanliness.

In 1796, Dr. Smith was accorded the distinction of election to the staff of New York Hospital. The following year he was listed with three physicians and four surgeons on the staff who were allowed to instruct students; of these he was the only one who had not received a medical degree. That the hospital corresponded in its aims and methods to those clinics established in postrevolutionary France can be inferred from a contemporary description: "The Medical student here learns the causes and symptoms of disease, observes their various types and characters, listens to the prescriptions of physicians, watches the operation of remedies administered, and notes events in each case."[17] Clearly New York Hospital followed the observation method and encouraged the physician's active participation in the practice of medicine.

Between his work at the hospital and his contacts with doctors throughout the Northeast and mid-Atlantic states via his editorship of *The Medical Repository*, Elihu Smith became active in the growing number of medical practitioners who remained loyal to the Republican cause that their profession had embraced at the time of the Revolution. He was a utopist—he completed 14 pages of a work in which he envisioned a "Utopia" in the newly opened Northwest Territory—a freethinker who renounced the Christian faith in which he had been raised, and a believer in the efficacy of reason to resolve human problems. Though he was not directly involved in the Philadelphia yellow fever controversy (because of his New York residency), he partook of every aspect of the national discourse that arose from the recurring epidemics.

Smith's major contribution to that discourse was a series of letters, written in 1795 and published a year later by Noah Webster, Jr., in which the young doctor discusses the *Fevers Prevalent in the U.S. for a Few Years Past.* In these letters Smith expressly discusses the 1795 yellow fever epidemic in New York and sets out his reasons for adopting the view that the fever was not imported but was the result of the unsanitary conditions that prevailed most particularly in the regions of the docks. The fourth letter is especially revealing: it deals with the immigrant inhabitants of the region who, Smith claims, were the principal sufferers in the epidemic. He shows them to be victims not only of the fever but also of poverty and oppression in this country equal to that which they had hoped to escape by emigrating.

In this letter Smith reverses the cause-and-effect relationship between the fever and the foreigners who were being blamed for its importation. In pointing to the sufferings of the immigrants as the main reason for their having emigrated, he was attempting to thwart the Federalist aim in linking disease and revolution. That connection was furthered by the insurrection in Santo Domingo, which brought to U.S. port cities (the principal sites of epidemic) many who were fleeing that disruption and who, because of their long exposure to yellow fever, gave the appearance of being immune when in fact they were simply able to resist infection. Irish immigrants too were subject to the linkage of disease and revolution, largely because of Ireland's steady resistance to England and also because the Irish gathered in great numbers in the ghettolike neighborhoods near the docks where the disease was most active. Because of the number of people confined in these neighborhoods, the fever spread quickly through them, feeding in turn the notion that the fever—like the violence and crime for which these districts were noted—had originated there. Given the conditions of the dock areas, it was no coincidence that the Democratic clubs flourished in them, under leaders who later used their experiences in the epidemics to gain greater participation in government.

During the 1795 epidemic in New York Smith "sat with the sick in every part of the city . . . ate with them . . . assisted and watched with them. . . . I have thought of nothing else, talked of nothing else, and written of nothing else than this same fever" (Cronin, 152). These experiences forced him to see, clinically, not only the bodily illnesses of his patients but the circumscribed area within the city, the immigrant ghetto—a space separate and distinct from its surroundings—where they lived. On 20 October, at the height of the epidemic, he recorded in his diary his climb up a hill from which he could survey this entire region. Concentrating on a particular area, "the lowest part of the city," he observes it closely, marking its boundaries, the types of buildings contained therein, the condition of its streets relative to water, sunlight, and air, the condition of the people who live there, and the prevailing winds off both the river and the land.

Smith's conclusion was that the source of the fever was not the inhabitants of this region but rather the conditions under which they lived. In his published letters on the subject the doctor puts forward his conviction that to continue to build cities in America as they had been is to doom the nation to pestilential disease "as fatal in America as in the old world."[18]

He offers a detailed plan of a model city, including suggestions for sewers, a fresh water supply, control of the waterfront warehouses, and so forth. What he terms "a rigid police," that is, a policing of sanitation, should be uniformly observed in all cities, he says, though he despairs of Philadelphia, which he believes "doomed to calamity": "The citizens will not believe the evil to arise among themselves and therefore must be left to their fate." He cannot resist, however, offering the environmentalist opinion that, "if all the cross streets and back houses in Philadelphia could be levelled and the ground converted into flower gardens and grass plots, the citizens would, in twenty years, celebrate the anniversary of their destruction, with as much fervor as the republicans in France celebrate the demolition of the Bastille" (*Papers*, 252).

Taken all in all, Smith's letters provide a stunning view into the conditions of inner-city life, as well as a spirited defense of the poor and immigrant populations of American cities. His opinions must have rankled the importationists, who would have quickly picked up on Smith's republican attitudes by his reference to the French Revolution and his talk of policing the cities for better sanitation. France, in the wake of the 1789 revolution, had passed numerous laws pertaining to medicine and public health and, in 1794, had created "health schools" in response to the grievous lack of physicians, most of whom had been turned out of their colleges of surgery the year before. The health schools, or clinics, were the foundation of the reform of medicine undertaken by the revolutionary government in the interests of the poor who could not afford medical care.

The similarity between the ideas of Elihu Smith and those of the government in France was the obvious result of his admiration for such republican reform movements. More interesting, though, is the similarity between his physical observation of the plague-ridden area of New York City, and the physician's gaze—of the diseased body and, by dissection, of the dead body—noted by Foucault. "Life, disease, and death now form a technical and conceptual trinity," Foucault writes about the restructuring of eighteenth-century medical thought (144); one commentator has schematized that triangle of medical perception by placing death at the point from which the medical gaze originates, so that life and death, both formerly obscured by the body itself, come into full view.[19] From the vantage point of the New York hilltop Elihu Smith was able to look into the diseased body of the city's poorest area and perceive, within the framework of his republican, environmentalist conviction, that the cause of yellow fever was poor sanitation.

From mapping out in words the areas where the disease was most prevalent it was but one step to the introduction of medical cartography in *The Medical Repository*. A map of the same area described in Smith's journal in

1798 was done by Dr. Valentine Seaman, Smith's friend and colleague at New York Hospital, who used it in his argument against the importation theory of yellow fever origin. It was the first use of a medical spot map in which an area was isolated not for quarantine, as in earlier times, but for study—to establish a relationship between disease and some other factor or factors within the area.[20]

It would be too great a loss to omit from this discussion of Smith's letters on the fever mention of one in which he relates that in mid-July 1795 (an epidemic year in New York), "clouds of musketoes, incredibly large and distressing," appeared in the city and stayed long after the time when they usually departed. "Almost every person suffered exceedingly from the bites of these insects," he writes, "and foreigners especially." The physical discomfort caused by "these animals," he concludes, "no doubt predisposed the well to be affected by the fever; while they extremely harrassed the sick, and retarded their recovery" (*Papers*, 76). Still so improbable was the idea of insects as vectors of disease that even while he considered every conceivable cause, Smith saw this onslaught as little more than "distressing." Ever true to his theory and his political beliefs, however, he sees the mosquitoes as having been troublesome to "foreigners especially," thus absolving once again the immigrant population on whom the Federalists blamed the epidemic.

What becomes obvious by tracing the development in America of the yellow fever discourse is the way in which it encompasses a bundle of related topics—rationalism, science, politics, economics, and other subsidiary interests. At the center of it all is the eighteenth-century physician, who by his gaze makes the diseased body an object of knowledge. But when the individual body failed to yield specific knowledge of the disease to which it was subject, as was the case with yellow fever, the next step was to consider the diseased as members of a group: the poor, the immigrants, the blacks. The coincidence of yellow fever epidemics in America with the emergence of a partisanship that extended to every aspect of social and political life furthered such collectivization; the ideas associated with revolutionaries, or with immigrants, or with blacks, were just as easily associated with yellow fever. In the attempt to deflect these associations the medical profession began to study space, and the groups within specific spaces, by structuring them—as in the use of spot maps—in the hope that the results of such study might overturn the view of America as a land disgraced by nature. Thus, in fact, did the movement toward the social sciences and the social experimentation of the nineteenth century begin in America.

It was against this use of scientific rationalism that Charles Brockden Brown set his romantic literature, in which he challenged what he later described as "the rage for explaining every thing" (*View*, 249n). By the time Brown used that phrase, he had come to terms with his anger at the medical profession and could openly question (though still with some emotion) both groups of yellow fever theorists on their accuracy and their motivations. And well he might, since neither side had been proven right and he had every reason to believe Smith was wrong.

Convinced of the correctness of his own position, the young doctor had assured Brown of the safety of his Pine Street neighborhood, and so, in the late summer of 1798 when Charles was visiting there and epidemic swept New York, the friends remained in the city while Smith saw fever patients day and night. They might have escaped the disease even so had it not been for the arrival of a fellow physician, Dr. Jean Baptiste Scandella, an Italian visiting in America who had attended a family stricken by the disease and himself fell ill. With nowhere to turn, he came to Dr. Smith and was taken into the household. Almost immediately both Smith and Brown contracted yellow fever, and in two days Smith was dead. Only Brown's swift removal to the Port Jervis home of the playwright William Dunlap saved his life.

By the middle of 1799 Brown already had in print *Arthur Mervyn*, the historical romance based on the Philadelphia yellow fever epidemic of that year. The book is his tribute to Elihu Hubbard Smith, a eulogy that echoes all of his friend's republican and environmentalist beliefs. If anything mars its sincerity it is the oft-noted opportunism of his hero, whose willingness to embrace causes that further his own interests has made him the subject of much critical comment. Arthur's opportunism becomes especially troublesome in light of Brown's association of the fever with the prevailing social illness, self-interest. These conflicted emotions, repressed in *Arthur Mervyn*, surface in the work that he produced almost simultaneously with it, *Edgar Huntly*. While he was still working on part 2 of Mervyn's story (published in 1800), Brown began the composition of *Edgar Huntly, or, Memoirs of a Sleep-Walker*. The similarity in title format signals the relationship between the two works, as does the mystery of the murdered friend that initiates the second tale, for if *Arthur Mervyn* is Brown's conscious, daytime memorial to Elihu Smith, *Edgar Huntly* is his unconscious, night-evoked rebuke of him.

As Elihu Hubbard Smith lay dying of yellow fever, Charles wrote to his own brother in Philadelphia, "My heart sickens at the perpetual recital to which I am compelled to be an auditor, and I long to plunge myself into woods and deserts where the faintest blast of rumor may not reach me."[21] In a sense he did plunge into woods and deserts in writing *Edgar Huntly*, the work that has become generally recognized as his best, and the one in which he allows the greatest freedom to his imagination.

= *Edgar Huntly, or, Memoirs* = of a Sleep-Walker

Charles Brockden Brown's avowed purpose in offering *Edgar Huntly* is often quoted. He states in his preface that such trappings of Gothic horror as were familiar from European romances were unsuited to the American writer; but he also notes that "America has opened new views to the naturalist and politician," and that "new springs of action, and new motives to curiosity should operate; . . . the field of investigation, opened to us by our own country, should differ essentially from those which exist in Europe."[22] Even allowing for the peculiarities of eighteenth-century diction, these words have a faintly clinical ring, their tone reinforced by Edgar Huntly's announcement, issued even before he begins his narrative: "What light has burst upon my ignorance of myself and of mankind! How sudden and enormous the transition from uncertainty to knowledge!" (Huntly, 6). Critics have been almost unanimous in pointing out the fatuousness of this exclamation given the ignorance of both himself and mankind that Huntly continues to exhibit to the end of his story. Nor is there any great clarity about the nature of the "knowledge" he claims to have gained, though the book is very much concerned with the acquisition of knowledge. Although the work has not been thus far seen in this manner, it seems likely that the "knowledge" Brown speaks of in grand, though vague, terms is in fact "science"—specifically, that medical science that had so drastically affected his life, and against which Brown sets his romance as an opposing view.

Edgar Huntly is a young Pennsylvanian whose friend, Waldegrave, has been mysteriously murdered. His body was left beneath a huge tree to which Huntly returns again and again in the hope of learning something of the murderer. On one such excursion, at midnight, he sees a man digging under the tree. Closer inspection reveals the man to be Clithero Edny, a recent immigrant from Ireland who works on a nearby farm. Edny is completely unaware of his actions at the time Huntly encounters him because he is sleepwalking. Huntly views this condition as an indication of guilt and is bent on determining its cause. He pursues Edny into the wilderness and eventually obtains from him the story, not of Waldegrave's murder, but of Edny's involvement in the affairs of a wealthy European family, of a murder he committed in England supposedly in self-defense, and of his attempt to murder his erstwhile patroness out of a misdirected sense of "pure benevolence." From all of these misadventures Edny has fled to the safety of America.

Huntly's compassion is aroused by the story, and soon he has begun to identify with Edny to such an extent that he himself sleepwalks, experiencing a sense of guilt much like that which he has observed in the man who has now become his alter ego. In his sleep, Huntly plunges into the Pennsylvania wilderness and wakes only after having fallen into a cave. Beginning with his experiences in the cave, there follows a series of adventures involving Lenape Indians, the rescue of a female held captive by them, numerous narrow escapes from death, and a final return home, where Huntly learns at last that Waldegrave was the victim not of Clithero Edny but of marauding "savages." In the course of these adventures Huntly appears to have acquired a new awareness of human nature by experiencing a side of himself he had never known. Despite this awareness, however, Huntly refuses to accept the word of others that Edny is insane and, through misguided benevolence, sets off a chain of events that allows Edny to make a second attempt on the life of his former patroness, now pregnant and living in New York. The attempt fails, but the woman miscarries as a result of the attack, and Huntly is left, at the story's end, with the knowledge of his own culpability.

Brown's announced intent, it should be recalled, was to make use of American materials in the creation of a Gothic tale. Indian hostility and "the perils of the western wilderness," he claims in his preface, are the stuff of American terrors. But these were not the only terrors being faced in America: what Brown represses in this tale is any overt reference to the yellow fever epidemics such as those that appear in *Ormond* and *Arthur Mervyn*. Perhaps because he was not yet ready to face the truth of what had occurred in New York in the late summer of 1798, Brown displaced his fears, and his anger, making their objects vaguely menacing Lenape "savages" and a perilous landscape.

The landscape, America's natural environment, is a terrifying venue in this tale. When Huntly enters upon his wilderness trek there is not a spot that does not hide some danger; he is repeatedly described as being on the "verge" of disaster in some form or another. The word appears 16 times in the course of Huntly's narrative, and the word *maze* is used 12 times. Since a maze is one of the oldest learning devices known to man, the combination of the two words serves to underscore how perilous the educational process was by which Americans were coming to know their natural environment. Other symbols of death abound, such as various places of containment—the pit, caves, and other tomblike enclosures that further support the suggestion of a dangerous environment. Locked chests and cabinets containing the secrets of dead persons give way, as the story continues, to larger images of death. One is a natural cliffside shelter, described as "somewhat resembling a coffin shape, and not much larger in dimensions" (*Huntly*, 217). Another is an oven in which Huntly seeks refuge. Both fail him: the oven collapses from his weight, and the narrowness of the shelter forces him to abandon it. Like Brown himself, Huntly survives, but the pattern of imagery points up a womb-tomb theme that culminates in the miscarriage of the unborn child and reveals the underlying subject of the book to have been death.

Although it is Huntly's trek through the labyrinthine wilderness that leaves the deepest impression on the reader, his reason for being in the wilderness is of even greater significance. Huntly himself seems not to under-stand his own motives, and in this the subtitle of the original piece from which *Edgar Huntly* derives, "Sky-Walk, or, The Man Unknown to Himself," is entirely appropriate. Nevertheless, in Brown's romances motivation as-sumes near-Jamesian proportions, and the question of Huntly's motivation is crucial to understanding Brown's repressed intention because of the conscious or unconscious parallel between Huntly's actions when confronted by a mystery and those of Elihu Smith in the face of the mysterious disease, yellow fever.

Clithero Edny, the Irish immigrant, is shunned by his Pennsylvania neighbors for his furtive behavior. But when Huntly, in his search for the murderer, demands and receives of Clithero his story, he is so moved by the Irishman's recital of Old World sufferings that he is immediately convinced of his innocence. Driven by his own fears, however, Edny disappears into the wilderness, only to be pursued by his confessor, who is determined to restore Edny's mind to a "tranquil and wholesome existence" (*Huntly*, 95). In other words, Huntly seeks to restore him to health. To find the object of his benevolence, Huntly is forced to follow the mazelike paths of what might be termed the "cave of the mind." During this journey his identification with Edny is so complete that he too becomes a sleepwalker; as in the unfortunate case of Elihu Smith, doctor and patient become identical in disease.

In effect, Brown refutes the local-origin theory through Huntly, the very theory he had expounded in *Arthur Mervyn*. The refutation of his friend Elihu Smith probably was too painful to execute overtly, especially when Smith had paid so dearly for his error; only covertly, it seems, in the guise of unconscious sleepwalking, could Brown contradict the doctor's word. His rebuttal extends even to a striking rejection of the cartographer's grid approach to landscape, by which the local-origin proponents had attempted to establish the fever's cause. As Huntly pursues Edny to the summit of a hill he is described as taking a circular direction, which only brings him back to the spot from which he set out. To gain a vantage point and view the full horizon, Huntly turns his attention to another, tunnel-shaped interior space. Having passed through the center of the cylinder to arrive at a second summit beyond, he slowly scans the horizon. As his eye travels over the landscape, which has about it, he claims, a "sort of sanctity and awe," he observes its every aspect and is startled by the sudden appearance in his field of vision of a human face. As he gazes its features gradually become recognizable and he exclaims, "Man! Clithero!" (*Huntly*, 105).

This acknowledgment of Clithero Edny has been seen by some as a healing of Huntly's psychic split, but the text does not support this since Huntly benefits not at all from the gesture. Instead he plunges into a participation in Edny's madness, and the winding paths along which Huntly follows his prey mirror the convoluted and tortuous turns of a diseased mind. Something other than Huntly's psychic healing seems to be involved in the acknowledgment of Edny's humanity. Huntly's ascent to the promontory from which he sights Edny is made by a series of circular turns. Once at its peak Huntly commands a view "more ample" than any he has hitherto enjoyed. Brown's description of the natural landscape his hero beholds is wildly romantic: "[A] chaos of rocks and precipices was subjected, at one view, to the eye"

(*Huntly*, 101). It is while he muses on the chaotic landscape that Huntly suddenly sees among the rocks Edny's melancholy countenance and cries out the acknowledgment of the immigrant as his fellow man.

This projection of the rationalist sensibility onto a natural landscape is the focal point of Brown's romantic statement. Moreover, in its circularity Brown's landscape—even if it is a phantasm of Huntly's distorted perception—is the antithesis of the geographic grid created by Dr. Seaman out of Elihu Smith's hilltop observations. Nor is the aim of the grid—to serve as an instrument by which to establish a connection between yellow fever and its cause—far from Brown's formulation. When Huntly recognizes the fugitive Edny, the man whom he would heal, he is "thrilled": "Horror and shuddering invaded me as I stood gazing upon him, and, for a time, I was without the power of deliberating on the measures which it was my duty to adopt for his relief" (*Huntly*, 105). In just such a manner had Dr. Smith gazed on the worst plague precinct in New York and deliberated on what measures it was his duty to adopt for the relief of its inhabitants. As Huntly struggles to arrive at the best remedy for Edny's ills, impulse drives him to call out and acknowledge the renegade's humanity.

The humanitarian motives of Elihu Smith and others who thought as he did are conveyed in Huntly's impulsive cry. But the doctor's inability to discern the partisan context within which the humanitarian "sees" things, or gains knowledge of them, is also depicted in the novel by Huntly's ignorance of his own motives and by the circularity of the landscape, which repeatedly brings Huntly back to his point of origin, that is, to his own perceptions. His original desire, to uncover the truth of his friend's murder, points to an even deeper motive—to explain away the mystery. Thereafter his perceptions of everything—of the landscape, of Edny—are shaped by this desire. Just as Brown denounced the medical discourse surrounding the yellow fever epidemics as "the rage for explaining everything," motivated by "the dogmatic spirit that imagines the causes of every thing within our reach" (*View*, 249n), in *Edgar Huntly* his hero despairingly exclaims, "Disastrous and humiliating is the state of man! By his own hands is constructed the mass of misery and error in which his steps are forever involved" (*Huntly*, 278).

By 1803, when he translated Volney's treatise, Brown could openly inveigh against rationalism for refusing to accept the element of mystery in human experience; but when he wrote *Edgar Huntly* he was not ready to do so. Then the experiences of the summer of 1798 were all too fresh, and Brown had to vent his anger and his grief at what he perceived as willful self-deception on the part of those Republican partisans who tied the local-origin theory of yellow fever to their political sentiments. Like Edgar Huntly, Elihu Smith had wandered through a maze of conflicting information on the fever, ever on the "verge" of falling over that precipice of ignorance that proved his undoing.

Seen in the context of the yellow fever controversy, which raged around the author at every point for at least five years and ultimately involved him in the most immediate, dire fashion, *Edgar Huntly*, already a critical success, gains historical importance and extends the meaning of its companion piece, *Arthur Mervyn*, by countering the local-origin theory expounded there. *Edgar Huntly* was the last of Charles Brockden Brown's romances. Brown had lost the stimulus that fed his imagination and called forth the fictional response through which he asserted his will—the prod of Elihu Smith's opposing views. What followed were two feeble attempts (both in 1801) at the senti-mental novel, *Clara Howard* and *Jane Talbot*. Thereafter, until his death in 1810, he turned to editing literary journals. Nevertheless, the romantic attraction to mystery—which Smith had labeled disease—survived in America, producing a literature of the type Alexis de Tocqueville had pre-dicted: "devoid of order, regularity, science, and art," but rich in the consider-ation of shadowed areas of human behavior.[23] As did each of Brown's other romances, *Edgar Huntly* helped prepare the way for that body of literature, not only by its psychological elements but by its attention to nature as a kind of "condition" with which Americans would have to learn to live.

Perhaps because of its appearance at a point in history when interest in science was accelerating, yellow fever, especially its epidemic appearance in the 1790s, is the best documented epidemical disease in America. Although outbreaks of other diseases may have been more devastating in terms of lives lost—by which measure the influenza epidemic of 1918 was certainly far worse—none has so threatened the political life of the nation. The yellow fever epidemics shook the newly laid philosophical foundations of the Republic, and the issues they aroused have never been entirely put to rest in the United States, as current events bear out. That yellow fever can yet serve, as it does in John Edgar Wideman's "Fever," as an image for the social ills of the nation attests to the inherent power of the idea of contagion in the United States. As Wideman demonstrates, the idea still needs only a climate of fear to cause it to be widely associated with minorities and others whose stories do not appear, for the most part, in history. These individuals are dependent upon literature to document the events of their lives and to point out the national tendency to view the victims of social ills as the cause.

4

The Disease of Poverty

EVEN THOSE AMERICANS WHO KNOW SOMETHING OF THE smallpox epidemics in colonial America or may have heard of the yellow fever epidemics that came later often know little or nothing of the three episodes of cholera in this country in 1832, 1849, and 1866. No literary piece speaks directly of the disease, as do Brown's and Hawthorne's of yellow fever and smallpox, though it may be that Hawthorne was moved to write "Lady Eleanore's Mantle" because of cholera's migration in 1832 from England to America. Walt Whitman, when he was writing fiction in the 1840s (and calling himself Walter), created a murderous character who redeems himself by becoming one of those "men and women, heedless of their own small comfort, who went out amid the diseased, the destitute, and the dying, like merciful spirits," during the cholera epidemic in New York City.[1] Later, in section 37 of "Song of Myself" (1855) Whitman projects himself into this image, becoming the all-comforting persona who identifies with the afflictions of all people:

Not a cholera patient lies at the last gasp
      but I also lie at the last gasp,
My face is ash-color'd, my sinews gnarl, away
      from me people retreat.
Askers embody themselves in me and I am embodied
      in them,
I project my hat, sit shame-faced, and beg.[2]

It is significant that Whitman, who was so conscious of all that went on in New York City, should make the connection between the cholera patient and poverty.

Edgar Allan Poe's "King Pest" (1835) and "The Masque of the Red Death" (1842) make no such concrete connections. Both allude to the epidemics, but so obliquely that the point of the allusions has been dulled for most readers by the lack of historical reference. Poe's tales offer interesting contrast in their approaches—one comic, one serious—to the same theme, but neither tells us anything about the epidemics in nineteenth-century America. Though it was not Poe's habit to make his stories specific to America, the absence of such reference in these two tales seems to reflect the same lacuna regarding cholera that exists generally in literature of the time.

= The "Foreign" Disease =

In part it is the decidedly unpleasant nature of the disease that makes it unsympathetic to artistic efforts. Cholera's progress is neither poetic nor picturesque, and unlike tuberculosis, it does not allow its victims to languish over a period of time; its onset is sudden and its course swift, with death occurring usually within hours of its first appearance. According to the historian Charles Rosenberg, however, the scope of the three nineteenth-century epidemics was large enough to have warranted more attention.[3] Thousands perished. How is it that Americans seem not to have consciously "seen" these epidemics, indeed, seem to have repressed much of the history of them? In telling the cholera story Rosenberg supplies a number of plausible answers to this question, but his chief argument can be summed up as follows: America did all in its collective power to distance itself from the disease by assuming the attitude that, since the disease was of foreign origin (unlike yellow fever, which was unknown outside the Western Hemisphere), it reflected nothing of the American experience, and that its victims were limited to those whose way of life invited such disaster. My discussion of the disease will consider the implications of each part of this argument—cholera's exoticism, and those who contracted it—before going on to the wider sociocultural dimensions of its absence from American literature.

Known as Asiatic cholera, the disease was historically associated with such countries as India and China and prior to the nineteenth century had not been known to appear in epidemic form outside of Asia. But early in that century it began to show its gruesome aspect in Europe, especially in France and England. With the heavy commerce and transport between these nations and the United States, it was inevitable that cholera should arrive in the New World as well, regardless of the feelings of Americans about its inappropriateness to their surroundings.

Cholera is a nasty disease, one that breeds in food and water tainted by bacterial organisms that thrive on sewage. It enters the intestines causing severe and sudden cramps, diarrhea, vomiting, fever, and dehydration. Because of the rapid and dramatic loss of bodily fluid, death can occur in a matter of hours or within a day, especially among children, the elderly, and the weak. The disease is contagious and infection usually occurs when substances contaminated by feces are ingested.

Set the nastiness of this disease, with its primary locus in the bowels, against the Jeffersonian ideal of the new Republic of virtue and one can begin to understand the reluctance of Americans to recognize its appearance in their midst. When cholera first struck the United States during the early years of the Jacksonian era, America was still a rural country whose healthy population could see nothing in its environment even remotely like those conditions that gave rise to the disease in the non-Christian nations (a psychologically powerful association for Americans) where it had been largely confined. It is interesting to speculate on the effect the first cholera epidemic may have had on the eventual abandonment of the idea, so vigorously promoted by Cong. Thomas Hart Benton of Missouri, of a northwest passage to the Orient. This dream dated from the era of European expeditions to the New World, and Jefferson revived it when he commissioned Meriwether Lewis and William Clark to find a route across the country to the Pacific Ocean so that the nation could open up commerce with the Orient. In the early decades of the nineteenth century fur traders and merchants of all kinds were eager for such commerce to begin, and from the time Lewis and Clark returned with news of a route along the Columbia River there was a great deal of talk in America about China, India, and "Asiatic" trade.

Thomas Hart Benton saw trade with the Orient as America's opportunity to establish commercial independence from England and Europe and continued to promote the idea until, in the 1840s, the country began to plan a transcontinental railroad and lost interest in the passage to India. There were many reasons for this turn of events, but one wonders if the association of cholera with the Far East played a part in making the nation less interested in further Asian contact. It is difficult to be certain that the connection was even strongly made between cholera and the Far East, since the disease entered the country with immigrants from Europe. These newcomers were flooding into America in such numbers that the eastern port cities, unable to accommodate them properly, were beginning to exhibit some of the same social conditions as those in Europe.

New York City, with its overcrowding and the resultant filth and crime, was a prime example. French, Irish, and German immigrants swelled the city's population and, as the medical historian John Duffy says, became "a constant factor in the health of New York."[4] Often they came off the boats sick with typhus or smallpox, and the conditions in which most of them were forced to live in the city soon brought on other ills. The better provisioned Germans could afford to move westward to the interior, but the Irish remained where they landed and became New York's slum inhabitants. Hogs and other animals shared the city's streets and homes with many of its human inhabitants, though only the animals may be said to have benefited from the heaps of garbage left to decompose in the streets and gutters. Drinking water was not fit to be called by that name and caused dysentery, and the contaminated meats from filthy butchering shops could only be made edible by masking both appearance and odor with thick gravies and pungent garlic. Families shared crowded living quarters with strangers to alleviate the cost of housing, and the poorest in the city dwelled below ground in wet, unfinished cellars. Graft and corruption at the political level kept major improvements from being realized, and the wealthy managed to ignore the worst aspects of city life by establishing an enclave of resorts along the East River and by building homes located safely beyond the city limits.

By this time the miasmatic theory of disease causation had taken firm hold in American medicine, and the environmental suppositions of Dr. Benjamin Rush and his followers, including Dr. Elihu Hubbard Smith, were accepted as fact. Which is not to suggest that these suppositions had been acted upon by responsible governmental agencies and an enlightened populace; only that there was a general agreement that clean air and water contributed greatly to good health, and a recognition that filth left in the streets and allowed to flow into the drinking water was dangerous. In rural areas water was obtained from wells dug on private property. In the cities some home owners maintained their own wells, often shallowly dug, but most city dwellers were dependent upon the private companies that sold barrels of water brought from country streams, which often were polluted, though the popular belief was that if water didn't smell bad, it was drinkable. Only the poorest in the cities drank from the city-supplied pumps, which provided entire communities with the foulest of water, usually contaminated by waste products.

The earlier practice of burying the dead in church graveyards located in the center of town was abandoned after the yellow fever epidemics. During the fever years in the 1790s, it had been impossible to keep up with the numbers of bodies needing burial; corpses were disposed of in mass interments in hastily dug pits. Later it was deemed too unhealthy to breathe the air of decomposition that arose from the centrally located graveyards, and early in the 1830s the first American cemeteries situated outside town limits were opened. In New York City another effect of the yellow fever epidemics was the establishment of a rudimentary board of health whose chief duty was to enforce quarantine laws during epidemics. Since the mayor functioned as head of the board, however, political and economic interests usually prevailed over medical concerns.

= A Disease of the "Lower Classes" =

In the summer of 1832 cholera came to New York, the first American city to experience the disease; the earliest recorded cases were members of a family of Irish immigrants (Rosenberg, 25). The disease quickly spread through the immigrant quarters and those of the lower classes and working poor. From there it moved to the lowest level of the city's inhabitants, the thugs and gang members of the Five Points section, the worst area in the city, where it was further spread by prostitutes. Rum, the favorite drink of the poor, became the most common medicine, for the most part self-administered since few of the city's doctors were willing to venture into the contaminated neighborhoods. As in the days of yellow fever, those who could, whether doctors or laymen, left the city. Those who remained prayed (though Pres. Andrew Jackson refused to declare a national day of prayer and fasting) and comforted them-selves with the "knowledge" that this filthy disease was limited to those who "were festering wounds in the face of society," as the *New York Mercury* reported on 2 August 1832. John Pintard, a prominent banker and founder of the New-York Historical Society, piously expressed his gratitude to God that the disease was "almost exclusively confined to the lower classes of intemperate dissolute & filthy people huddled together like swine in their polluted habitations"; how much worse, he shuddered, if it were to occur among the city's "regular householders" (Rosenberg, 42).

The epidemic ended with the summer; the "regular householders" were not much worse for the onslaught and some of the city's most offensive citizens had been "providentially" removed. Almost 20 years went by without further signs of the dread disease. As the decade of the 1840s drew to an end, however, Europe was engulfed by revolution and cholera. In 1849 a ship arrived in New York carrying over 300 persons some of whom were already dead of cholera, others of whom were ill, and all of whom had been exposed to it. The epidemic that ensued was worse than that in 1832, and doctors were even more confounded by it.

Medical discourse of the period reveals the same kind of confusion that prevailed during the yellow fever epidemics, for neither disease seemed obvi-ously contagious. Not everyone who was in contact with the sick became ill, not everyone living in the affected sections of the city fell victim to the disease, and though cholera showed a tendency to occur in various parts of the city at approximately the same time, it seldom occurred in the better neighborhoods. Though the nonmedical population most at risk scoffed at the doctors' refusal to accept the fact that the disease was contagious, it was this last factor, the absence of cholera in the better neighborhoods, that prevailed in the thinking of a majority of the people in New York, medical and lay. According to their logic, only the disreputable members of society fell victim to cholera, those guilty of the sin of poverty, from which followed, in the moralistic thinking of most Americans of the time, all the worst sins of humankind. As Rosenberg says, "By 1849, the connection between cholera and vice had become almost a verbal reflex. The relationship between vice and poverty was a mental reflex even more firmly established" (120). Strong sanitary measures eventually undertaken in New York City did much to alleviate the threat of cholera, but it is the economic relationship referred to by Rosenberg, and the moral perception that strengthened it, that is key to understanding America's reaction to cholera.

= The Disease of Poverty =

During the first two cholera outbreaks, disease per se was not much on the public mind; attention was focused instead on what was perceived as its cause—namely, poverty, which in turn was viewed as a vice. The contagion of this condition, seen as a moral failing, was more feared than cholera, for its consequences were neither of short duration nor confined to one societal level. Poverty was no longer tolerated as it had been in colonial America, when it was believed to be a necessary part of the human condition: "[I]n all times some must be rich, some poor," the Puritan leader John Winthrop declared in "A Model of Christian Charity" (1630). The needs of the new nation in the early decades of the nineteenth century called for a steady and industrious work force, and the nation's democratic philosophy held that in this New World of freedom no one need go without work and the benefits of one's own labor. Yet there was poverty in the United States, caused for the most part by the inability of the existing workplaces to absorb the large numbers of immigrants, most of whom were from agricultural countries and therefore not suited to working in the factories that were a major source of employment in the United States. Then, too, abuse of their newfound freedom led many immigrants into the worst of habits; alcoholism was a leading cause of impoverished families. Crime did exist, hand in hand with poverty and alcoholism and laziness and all the problems that accompany the kind of social upheaval represented by immigration rates that caused a trebling of the nation's urban population in the decade from 1820 to 1830. Strained by the cost of providing public assistance to the poor while at the same time having to pay high prices for goods to meet the high wage demands of skilled workers who knew they were in short supply, and (after the 1832 cholera epidemic) fearful of the havoc the poor were capable of spreading through the middle class, America began to look for answers to the problems of poverty and crime.

The first question that needed to be addressed echoed a similar medical question about the source of illness in the body: was it an internal or an external problem? That is, did the vice of poverty and its concomitant, crime, originate within the individual or was it caused by some external environmental factor? The answer arrived at in Jacksonian America was decidedly in favor of internal causation. Since the root of the problem lay within the deviant individual, the one who simply did not follow the same path as the majority, it was thought necessary to remove that individual from society for a period of indoctrination in religious principles and the all-important work ethic. This idea of separation from society, which had its origins in the quarantine used to isolate those contaminated by disease, gained credence during the nation's early experiences of epidemic diseases and informed its first experiment in social engineering, the penitentiary system in which prisoners were isolated, often from each other. As the reformist mentality coming out of New England took hold nationally between 1820 and 1860, quarantine, in the form of isolation, reeducation, and reform, gradually became the method of treatment for many forms of social deviance.[5] Cholera no doubt was the most obvious, and frightening, example of the deleterious effect the poor and criminal elements could have on the larger society and would have served as prime motivation to the reformers had their objectives been more medical than social.

= Poe's Allegories of Pestilence =

Three years after the 1832 cholera epidemic in New York, Edgar Allan Poe (then a resident of Baltimore) created one of his earliest and best literary burlesques out of an imagined incident during London's fourteenth-century bubonic plague. "King Pest, A Tale Containing an Allegory," is a spoof of the allegorical tales that Poe found so objectionable for their moralizing. His "heroes," two drunken sailors who violate the quarantine laws of the city by entering a forbidden area, stumble into the dais-chamber of the palace of King Pest the First, all of whose royal companions bear titles that in some way refer to pestilence. The king demands that the sailors join them in drinking a toast on bended knee to the prosperity of their Kingdom of Death. One of the sailors refuses to drink, while the other declares he will not bend the knee to one whom he recognizes as "Tim Hurlygurly the stage-player." A general brawl results during which one sailor is dumped into a hogshead of ale. His companion pushes King Pest through an open trap door, upsets the hogshead from which his liberated comrade tumbles sneezing, and both run off through the streets of London, carrying with them two ladies from the Court of Death. Despite the gruesome reality behind this farce, the story provokes laughter as Poe manages to poke fun at a number of moralistic attitudes, especially those that associated pestilence with drunkenness and ruffians such as sailors, ladies of the evening, and actors.

In 1842 Poe published his now critically acclaimed "Masque of the Red Death," an elaborately wrought and serious meditation on a pestilence whose "Avatar," or manifestation, was blood. Very likely Poe took the idea for his story from an account given in an 1832 letter written by the German romantic poet Heinrich Heine, which received wide quotation. Heine tells of a masked ball given in Paris in March 1832 where one of the harlequin-attired guests suddenly collapsed with symptoms of cholera. Soon after other guests were hurried to the Hôtel Dieu, where they died and were hastily buried, still wearing their domino costumes.[6]

Modern editors and anthologists often change "Masque" in the title of Poe's tale to "Mask," thus violating the author's allusion to the dramatic entertainments of Prospero, Shakespeare's poet-magician in *The Tempest*. Poe's Prospero, the prince in his tale, gathers a thousand of his courtly followers for a palatial masque at the very time that pestilence is devastating his kingdom. Such masques were especially grand in sixteenth- and seventeenth-century England, where they had mythological or allegorical themes. Here, then, is the companion piece to "King Pest," not a burlesque but a true allegory of heedless detachment from the death that stalks the kingdom.

Poe employs the architectural imagery that works so well for him elsewhere, such as "The Fall of the House of Usher" (1840). Like Shakespeare's, his Prospero also retreats, not to an island but to an abbey of his own design with an imperial suite of seven rooms. Each room, in the language implied by the prince's Italianate name, is a stanza, as in poetic form. The stanzas, or rooms, are color-keyed to varying emotions; the last room is a velvety violet of oblivion. In these rooms the prince entertains his thousand guests. The allegorical "poem" Poe contrives for his depiction of the palace is richly colorful and full of a sumptuous beauty that enraptures and provides security from the Red Death that walks without.

Like Spenser and his *Faerie Queene*, Poe's allegory is decidedly medieval in that it draws on the Dance of Death theme of the late Middle Ages.[7] The figure of Death, clad in grave shrouds and mask, appears at the entertainment and is taken for a reveler who has chosen for the occasion a singularly inappropriate costume. Insulted by this attire, which would remind those present of the world outside the palace, the prince pursues the guest into the seventh room, where the figure turns and confronts his host, who falls dead. When the revelers rush the shrouded figure they find no tangible form beneath his robe. "And now," Poe says, "was acknowledged the presence of the Red Death."[8]

As an allegory of the determined effort made by most nineteenth-century Americans (especially those wealthy enough to seek a place of retreat) to deny the cholera in their midst, the story works quite well, except for the fact that the disease did not reach into the upper levels of American society and therefore never forced an acknowledgment of its presence. It remained, in the cities at least, an affliction of the poor, who were easily dismissed from sight, so easily that they do not enter into Poe's conception. Even stripped of its historical referent, however, Poe's "Masque" is striking and makes a vivid impression on the mind. But because the author has deliberately chosen an ahistorical setting, the tale remains divorced from its contemporary context and thus fails to heighten our awareness of cholera in America. By "masking" his subject Poe in fact contributes to the collective blindness of his countrymen.

= Cholera and Literature =

Understanding the cholera story from a cultural perspective involves a great deal more than apprehending the facts and figures of the epidemics. In truth, it requires a study wider than what has been undertaken here, one involving an exploration of the social conditions not only in the cities, where the epidemics took their greatest toll, but beyond, into the regions of contemporary social engineering (of which the penitentiary system was but a part), which must be viewed as part of the nation's response to contagious diseases and to what was perceived as their sources—poverty and the crime it breeds. The reticence of American writers to render these concerns and themes into imaginative literature has robbed us of the opportunity to enter affectively into this side of the nineteenth-century democratic experience. That the most vivid account of poverty and homelessness in American literature of the time appears in Melville's *Redburn* (1849) and is set in Liverpool, England, says a great deal about the ability of American writers to enter into a form of national denial with regard to social problems in their own country.

It may be, however, that works such as *The Scarlet Letter* and *Moby-Dick* were influenced to some degree by their authors' awareness of the ease with which Americans, especially those nurtured on allegorical readings of the Bible, made mental associations of the sort that could so firmly link cholera with vice, and vice with poverty. More than any of its other characteristics, it is the mysterious nature of an epidemic that creates an atmosphere highly susceptible to multiple references and multiple interpretations. Though neither *The Scarlet Letter* nor *Moby-Dick* makes any reference to epidemical disease, the subjects of both are surrounded with a high degree of mystery. Verbal and mental correlations to the subjects are formed and communicated in both works, and associations of evil and guilt projected onto humans and other objects in nature. And in both works such correlations are made to seem highly questionable; indeed, the focus of *The Scarlet Letter* is on the ability of Hester Prynne to reorder the cognitive associations to the *A* she is forced to wear.

Works of literature must also be understood as much for what they do not say as for what they do—especially when a specific subject matter is being purposely ignored. Hawthorne's sensitive depiction in *The Scarlet Letter* of the effects of punitive isolation is set in Puritan New England, but it clearly is informed by contemporary social attitudes toward deviancy, which he well may have been addressing. Denial, avoidance, and slant reference are all part of the cholera story in America, a story left untold, for the most part, because of a sense of delicacy and because it was not supposed to happen in the New World.

5

The Disease That "Rides Mankind"

EVEN AS YELLOW FEVER WAS RETREATING TO THE SOUTHERN regions of the United States, routed in part by the clearing of land for new cities—among them the city of Washington, D.C.—another scourge was beginning to manifest itself in the nation. Charles Brockden Brown survived the yellow fever epidemics of the 1790s only to die at 39 (in 1810) of tuberculosis, and his was by no means an extraordinary case. By 1830 tuberculosis was a prime cause of death in America. That it was not understood to be a contagious disease contributed greatly to its high death rate, but it was principally lack of knowledge about the tubercle bacillus that allowed the disease to spread unchecked within the rapidly growing population. Even when the knowledge came, with the discovery in 1882 by the German scientist Robert Koch of the tubercle bacillus, efforts to apply it therapeutically were frustrated for many more years.

Tuberculosis, or consumption, as it was more commonly known, was not peculiar to America, nor was its appearance here and in Europe in the nineteenth century its initial global manifestation. History provides evidence of it in skeletons of ancient Egyptians, in descriptions of the illness by Roman historians, and in the varying treatments offered by physicians from the first-century Greek physician Galenus, who prescribed rest and underground residence, to seventeenth-century England's Thomas Sydenham, who sent his consumptive patients off on daily, galloping horseback rides.

Sydenham's treatment calls to mind Susan Sontag's point in her study *Illness as Metaphor* (1978) that in both English and French the disease is said to "gallop," so rapid can its progress be.[1] The title of this chapter, however, alludes not to this but to Ralph Waldo Emerson's "Ode, Inscribed to W. H. Channing" (1846), in which he derides the rampant consumerism of nineteenth-century America:

> 'Tis the day of the chattel,
> Web to weave, and corn to grind;
> Things are in the saddle,
> And ride mankind. (Whicher, 439)

Henry David Thoreau expressed much the same feeling, though directed toward the railroad, when he said, "We do not ride on the railroad; it rides upon us."[2]

The parallel between the consumption of "things" by the restlessly acquisitive Americans of Emerson's time and the consumption of the body by the tubercle bacillus will be clarified in the ensuing discussion of various works of American literature having to do with the disease. The literature reveals a general economic concern that suggests a desire—not unlike that of scientists working to connect diseases with their causes—to understand how economics influences a society. But the desire to understand the connection takes a romantic turn, as did many of the health practices of the time. Phrenology, the pseudoscience of reading skull configurations for signs of health and personality; Grahamism, the health teachings of Sylvester Graham, originator of the graham cracker; pathognomy and physiognomy, which claimed, respectively, that personality was revealed through body movement and through facial features; and a variety of theories on human sexuality; all flourished in nineteenth-century America while scientific research languished. Environmentalism, the belief that most disease was caused by airborne pollution, retained a firm grip on American medical thought, but cholera had roused a consciousness of the interplay between disease and poverty that proved troubling.

The connections between poverty and a disease such as cholera were obvious, to the nineteenth-century way of thinking: the poor were poor because of their dissolute way of life, which included crime and, inevitably, disease. Tuberculosis was another matter. The disease pervaded American society at all levels throughout the century, but little or nothing was known of its cause or treatment. The mystery surrounding the illness, and the fact that it did not spare even the "best" and most promising in American society, appears to have wakened an unacknowledged fear that the industrialization based on human and machine labor, which was fast becoming the very basis of America's economy, was in some way humanly enervating. Further, the pervasiveness of tuberculosis seems to have suggested to many, in an almost unconscious, subliminal way, the developing societal ills of an unbridled economy based on the profit motive. Initially, Emerson's generation attempted to deal with these ills metaphysically by urging a greater realization of spiritual power; but as the century wore on transcendental speculations on the nature of the world order gave way to a greater understanding of natural law. Still later, the application of social Darwinism to human society was countered by attacks on the superstructure of wealth and privilege that industrialization had wrought. Tuberculosis then became a target of the progressive reform movement, which viewed it as a product not only of unsanitary living conditions but of economic exploitation.

In the above excerpt from his "Ode," the tangible nature of Emerson's "things" in the saddle combines with his paradoxical image of the human as beast of burden to vividly depict the inversion of values the poem decries. According to the hierarchy of values set forth by Emerson, and by New England transcendentalism generally, spirituality enjoyed the highest rank; hence the consuming of material objects was demeaning to the spirit. "Spirit" and "matter," opposing forces throughout centuries of philosophic and religious thought, became values-laden terms, just as "sick" and "well" are value-laden signs. Usually, "wellness" indicates health, wholeness, even holiness (in the Teutonic origins of the word *health*), whereas "sickness"—and "disease" even more so—indicates a deviation from the norm of health. Faced with an epidemic of tuberculosis, Americans felt the need to legitimize, even spiritualize, the disease and to raise it to a plane of higher value; hence the consuming of the body, matter, that occurs in the progress of the disease became an experience endowed with spiritual value, in essence a spiritual empowering of the tubercular. Given the high incidence of tuberculosis in nineteenth-century New England, it is small wonder that in that region the desire to transcend matter became the basis of a philosophy. Indeed, the "economy" to which TB was literarily tied early in the century was an economy based on spiritual values, the attainment of which the disease was seen to facilitate. At the end of the century Henry James picked up on this peculiar economy and created a heroine, an American tubercular, who suffers not only from the disease but from a surfeit of spirituality.

James was reacting specifically to New England romanticism and its spiritualization of tuberculosis, as well he might. No similar attempt at spiritualization accompanied epidemics of yellow fever or cholera in this country. But tuberculosis struck with particular force in the New England states; any consideration of tuberculosis in America, therefore, must pay heed to its influence on the thinking of this formative region, especially given the philosophical thrust toward individual spiritual power over matter that developed there. One *might* even be led to consider Emerson's famous "transparent eyeball" experience as a moment of fevered excitation brought on by the tuberculosis that for years smoldered in his chest, though as we shall see, Thoreau's *Walden* speaks more to the point of spiritualized power.

= Tuberculosis Returns to America =

The rising incidence of tuberculosis in Europe and America in the nineteenth century was indicative of the peak-and-plateau cycle typical of many contagious diseases. Anything but galloping in its epidemic sequence, the disease is peculiar for the slowness with which it curves through its cycle; medical evidence suggests that the last epidemic period began as early as the seventeenth century, only reaching its peak in the midnineteenth century, by which time it had claimed millions. Contributing to the mortality figures were the rapidly changing conditions in society that accompanied this epidemic curve and intensified its effects. All the evils of modern industrialized societies conspired to aid the spread of tuberculosis, and though it is no respecter of rank or social status, economic factors became an integral part of its history. Only in 1945 was a cure found, in one of the so-called "miracle drugs," streptomycin, which was followed by other drugs equally effective in restoring health to a tubercular patient. At present the treatment involves two antibiotics, isoniazid and rifampin, taken in combination for a period of months.

Now, less than five decades after the discovery of a cure, this dread disease threatens to become epidemic once again. This time the cause is not a periodic upswing in the cyclical curve, but rather social factors actually present in the United States and at least potentially present in other nations. U.S. health officials reported a 5 percent increase nationally in tuberculosis cases in 1989 over the previous year. New York City has experienced the greatest jump in figures, with a reported 38 percent increase in 1990 over the previous year. The upsurge is most directly attributable to the AIDS epidemic (discussed in chapter 6), but it also has much to do with drug abuse, homelessness, extreme poverty among great numbers of our population, and a shift in immigration patterns that has brought to the United States individuals from nations where tuberculosis is still a primary killer. Some of the very factors, such as homelessness and drug abuse, that contribute to the growing epidemic also work against the ability of the medical profession to treat patients effectively: not all of the victims will seek medical help or follow through with the requisite lengthy course of treatment. In New York City steps have already been taken to hospitalize recalcitrant patients against their will and hold them until completion of a full course of treatment. (The law that permits this dates to 1915 when a New Yorker, Mary Mallon, known as "Typhoid Mary," was permanently committed to an isolation ward after infecting at least 50 people with typhus.)

Younger doctors often have had difficulty in even recognizing the insidious threat posed by TB, since many have never encountered the disease during their training and have been lulled into a false sense of security by an infrequency of reported cases. In fact, these two elements may have played into one another: doctors may not have been reporting cases of tuberculosis because they did not recognize it. (The same difficulty in diagnosing syphilis, unknown to many doctors who are now faced with the strongest reemergence of that disease in a half-century, is further complicated by the ability of syphilis symptoms to mimic those of many other diseases.) The dangers of misdiagnosis are especially devastating in tuberculosis: first, because the patient who is allowed to remain in the community is a constant risk to others; and second, because a misdiagnosis often results in treatment with types and quantities of medication not effective against the disease but capable of rendering the TB germs invulnerable to further drug therapy.

The sudden resurgence of tuberculosis has jogged medical and governmental agencies into activities they had not thought it was necessary to continue, such as mass education efforts, testing of groups and individuals believed to have been exposed, screening of immigrants from certain Third World countries, and a return to testing for the disease before allowing children to enter the public school systems of some large northeastern cities where newly arrived immigrants make up large portions of the population. These hurried and often agitated responses, especially on the part of governmental agencies (some of which have even pursued infected individuals into drug hangouts and abandoned buildings to press treatment upon them), indicates something of the seriousness accorded this disease.

= Mycobacterium Tuberculosis Humanis =

The bacterium whose nomenclature bespeaks its association with humankind is really part of a large family of bacteria of which only one other plagues the human race—leprosy. Mycobacterium tuberculosis humanis is a very small, rod-shaped organism dependent upon oxygen for survival and best adapted to a dark, moist environment. It reproduces slowly, but its virulence allows it to take its time; housed within a human host whose life span by comparison is infinitely shorter, it can reproduce itself to the point of overwhelming its host's defenses within a month. These defenses are principally the white blood cells, which attack the tubercle bacilli but may not be capable of stemming the tide, in which case the bacilli spread to lymph and circulatory systems and take up residence in the organs. Depending upon which organ is invaded (the liver, for one, is lethal to this bacilli), reproduction continues. The brain and the end points of the body's long bones provide a safe harbor, but the apices of the lungs, where oxygen levels are high, are especially nurturing, making this the most vulnerable region of the body and giving rise to the popular image of tuberculosis: the cough-ridden patient.

There are some strange aspects of the tubercle bacillus: some bacilli are relatively harmless; many people harbor the tiny rods within their bodies but manage to fight off the infection without becoming ill or infecting others; sometimes the disease becomes active, the patient is cured, but the bacilli reactivate years later. For those not able to withstand the initial invasion of virulent bacilli, and whose lungs are affected, lung tissue liquefies under the bacilli assault and seemingly consumes itself, hence the name consumption. As this happens, a larger area is made available to the invading bacilli, which quickly fill it up. The patient now presents the classic appearance of the TB sufferer: he or she coughs, with increasing constancy as the disease progresses, loses weight, and has a fever that rises in the late afternoon and falls at night but produces drenching night sweats. After a time blood vessels in the affected tissue rupture and then the sputum produced by the cough contains blood. There is a fatigue that alternates, without apparent cause, with excitement—often agitation—and in some cases there is pain in the chest cavity. A patient who has reached this stage will die if untreated, either directly from the TB in the lungs or from the failure of another vital organ similarly attacked. He or she has been the most dangerous to others at the time of coughing, when the bacilli are released into the air ready to be inhaled by another host.

Given the bleakness of this condition it is not hard to understand why governmental agencies would take an active part in preventing the spread of this disease. But government only entered the picture in the last decade of the nineteenth century, though tuberculosis had reached its peak in America about 1860. The turning point came, of course, with the discovery in 1882 that the disease was caused by bacteria and hence was infectious. Difficult though it is for us to accept, prior to this discovery TB was not believed to be a contagious disease, even while it was devastating the nation. When individuals contracted the illness they were often treated at home and directly nursed by numerous family members, from a sickbed located in the room most commonly occupied by the family. This would have been the room in which the central fireplace was located, and in the winter doors and windows would have been sealed to conserve the heat. Family members, sick and well, coughing or not, shared these quarters for most of the day during the winter months, even taking meals there. Henry David Thoreau, when he was dying from TB, made a point of having his meals with the family so as not to be "unsociable."

The lack of recognition of the threat presented to the family and to the community by the tubercular patient allowed the development of what can only be described as, in Susan Sontag's term, a mythology. The myth grew largely out of observations made of TB sufferers whose disease had settled in the lungs, since this was the most common site of infection and its symptoms there were more easily recognized than when it affected the brain, bones, or other organs. Even as late as 1938 the illness that killed Thomas Wolfe, author of *You Can't Go Home Again* (1940) and *Look Homeward, Angel* (1929), was not recognized as tuberculosis of the brain. To understand this less familiar aspect of the disease it will be useful to ignore chronology and examine its progress in Wolfe's life.

= Thomas Wolfe =

The onset of Thomas Wolfe's illness coincided with his entrance into Harvard in the fall of 1920. His undergraduate career at the University of North Carolina at Chapel Hill had been marked by considerable success in playwriting and philosophy, and his professors had urged graduate studies. His earlier plan to attend Harvard resurfaced, but his parents were unwilling to continue paying for his education. Young Tom struck a bargain with his mother by which he borrowed on an expected inheritance from his father, who was dying of cancer. They agreed to a year's tuition, and in September Wolfe was on his way north. On the train he contracted a cold that did not lessen in intensity after his arrival in Cambridge. In a letter to his mother, Wolfe described the progress of the disease and his feelings of dread:

> The thing got down into my chest and a week or two ago, I began to cough—at first a dry cough—then a rattling, tearing, sort of cough, full of phlegm. I became worried. My right lung was sore. . . . One night I started coughing here, in my room, and I put my handkerchief to my mouth. When I drew it away there was a tiny spot of blood on it. I was half sick with horror and I tried not to think of it. . . . The cold got better, the cough subsided, it has gone now—and the soreness has disappeared from my lung. But that is not the important thing; when this happened—which, I think, meant little—I saw the sure destruction . . . of my dreams and my poetry—and myself—and I couldn't face it.[3]

After this episode Wolfe frequently had racking colds that prostrated him with fever and sweats. One such cold occurred while he was traveling abroad in 1925, and in England he may have received a medical warning about the state of his lungs (Nowell, 95). In 1937 "a touch of the flu," as he described it, laid him low long enough that he sought medical care, after which he showed evidence of great agitation for a time until, having executed a new will, he seemed better in mind and body. It was, however, but the prelude to what was to come in the following year, when Wolfe undertook a western trip on one of the streamlined trains that commanded so much attention in the 1930s. At Seattle he impulsively decided to continue on to Vancouver, British Columbia, by steamship. On board, a fellow passenger was ill enough to catch Wolfe's attention; the writer offered him a drink of whiskey—straight from the bottle—and then drank from it himself. Wolfe contracted whatever respiratory disease his traveling companion had, and within 24 hours it turned to pneumonia. The author had entered upon his final illness.

Tests at a Seattle hospital were inconclusive: no tubercle bacilli were evident, but X-rays showed "a large area of consolidation in the right upper lobe, involving one-third to one-half of the right lung" (Nowell, 426). Some of the doctors involved in making the diagnosis refused to see in this evidence of TB, calling it instead an unresolved pneumonia. The spot on the lung responded to treatment, and plans were made for the patient's release from the hospital. By this time, however, Wolfe had begun to complain of severe and unremitting headache. Once again he appeared to respond to treatment and was allowed to leave the hospital. Wolfe attempted to settle into a Seattle apartment with his sister acting as nurse, but he was soon too weak to remain out of hospital. An examination indicated brain surgery for the suspected tumor or abscess, and he was sent by train to Johns Hopkins Hospital in Maryland. The long train ride almost killed him, and there were times when he lapsed into delirium.

The trephining (a procedure in which a circular section of bone is removed from the skull) performed at Johns Hopkins to relieve the pressure on the brain was ostensibly preparatory to further X-ray studies of the organ, but the procedure itself revealed, in the fluid that spurted from his skull, that Wolfe had tuberculosis of the brain. A last desperate effort to save his life through surgery was thwarted by the discovery that his brain was covered with bacilli. The "cold" that had so terrified him when he was first at Harvard was in fact tuberculosis of the right lung, and when the lesion healed over the tubercles were sealed inside. When he became ill with pneumonia in Seattle, the lesion opened and the tubercles entered his bloodstream, eventually settling in his brain (Nowell, 438). Within a week of the aborted surgery Thomas Wolfe was dead.

How far removed from the myth of the tubercular was the disease that destroyed Thomas Wolfe's brain and life can be judged from the absence of any wasting away of his body. The disease had healed itself in his lung, sparing him from the prolonged devastation that occurs in pulmonary tuberculosis. In another regard, however, there is a notable similarity between the author's silence on the subject of his illness (notable especially in a literary output made up almost exclusively of autobiographical novels) and that of other American writers who have been afflicted with tuberculosis. The outpouring of emotion and the acknowledgment of terror at the prospect of an early death that Wolfe shared with his mother in the letter quoted above never appeared in his novels. The closest he came to putting these feelings to literary use is in the masterful description of the death of the hero's brother, Ben, in *Look Homeward, Angel.*

The character is based on Wolfe's own brother, Benjamin Harrison, who is believed to have had pulmonary tuberculosis in childhood. He survived this illness but with the usual problem of "weak lungs," which made him highly susceptible to the influenza epidemic of 1918. Ben died in the fall of that year, when the second wave of the flu epidemic caught even President Woodrow Wilson and nearly brought to a halt the country's war effort. In *Look Homeward, Angel* Wolfe tells of Ben's body seeming to grow rigid in its death throes:

> But suddenly, marvelously, as if his resurrection and rebirth had come upon him, Ben drew upon the air in a long and powerful respiration; his gray eyes opened. Filled with a terrible vision of all life in the one moment, he seemed to rise forward bodilessly from his pillows without support—a flame, a light, a glory—joined at length in death to the dark spirit who had brooded upon each footstep of his lonely adventure on earth; and, casting the fierce sword of his glance with utter and final comprehension upon the room haunted with its gray pageantry of cheap loves and dull conscience and on all those uncertain mummers of waste and confusion fading now from the bright window of his eyes, he passed instantly, scornful and unafraid, as he had lived, into the shades of death.[4]

The passage exhibits the intensity of Wolfe's emotions, presumably evoked at the death of his own brother, as well as something of the fear he carried within (like the bacilli sealed only for a time within his lung), and the hope that he himself would meet death in so undaunted a manner.

= Romantic Tuberculosis =

It was pulmonary tuberculosis that provided the nineteenth century with its tubercular mythology, embodied in the ethereal sufferer too spiritual for the mundane world who is further refined by the disease. Strangely, tuberculosis evidently was perceived as a natural consumption of the body through which the body was spiritualized. Such romantic victims of the disease as the English poets Keats and Shelley and the composer Chopin lent credence to the myth, and the figure of the wan tubercular youth began to make its appearance in popular literature and on the stage. In both England and America— especially in New England, where climatic conditions made the disease particularly prominent—consumption came to be associated with artistic creativity and could lead critics, as in the case of Tom Moore, the sentimental Irish poet whom America took to its heart during his stay here, to crown with success some inferior efforts. The persistence of this view can be gauged by the almost mystical import attached by some critics to the one poem of true value produced by Sidney Lanier, a southern poet of the 1860s and 1870s. Occasionally one still finds a reference to "Sunrise," a poem written shortly before Lanier's death in 1881 from tuberculosis, as a product of the fevered animation of his elevated temperature. The disease seems to have been associated with creativity more in the popular mind, however; the transcendentalists were groping toward an understanding that was more inclusive and more spiritually empowering.

= Ralph Waldo Emerson =

Because climate was believed to be the major cause of "lung fever," English sufferers were sent to warmer regions, Italy especially, and New Englanders went to southern states, Puerto Rico, or the West Indies. In 1826 Ralph Waldo Emerson, then 23 and a divinity school graduate, set off on a southern journey, having had to abandon his first attempt at teaching because of his poor health. He had already experienced serious illnesses while at Harvard, but in 1826 he developed symptoms of tuberculosis. Two of his brothers, Charles and Edward, had been forced to alter their vocational plans for the same reason, and both left Concord at varying times in search of full recovery. Edward died of tuberculosis in 1834, and Charles died two years later; a third brother, William, was afflicted but recovered. Still another brother, John, who was born in 1799, had died of the disease when only seven, and it is possible that his illness, in the close confines of a large household (all the succeeding sons were born within the seven years of John's brief life), had tragic consequences for others in the Emerson family. The father died five years later at only 43, having suffered lung hemorrhaging, and his sons entered on their own dismal roads of tubercular illness.

Emerson's 1826 southern journey took him first to Charleston, South Carolina; but the winter there was too cold, and he considered going on to the West Indies. Eventually he settled on Florida. His journal entries for that winter describe his bodily ills, the "oppressions and pangs, chiefly by night," and "a certain stricture on the right side of the chest, which always makes itself felt when the air is cold or damp, and the attempt to preach or the like exertion of the lungs is followed by an aching."[5] The following spring he was able to preach an occasional sermon, but he noted—using the same image as in the later "Ode . . . to W. H. Channing"—that he was "still saddled with the villain stricture and perhaps he will ride me to death" (Rusk, 123). Surprisingly, Emerson recovered from TB and, though he was never in robust health, seems not to have suffered relapses.

Emerson's recovery from tuberculosis would not necessarily have indicated to him a lack of spirituality, but his Calvinist heritage caused him constantly to reprove and chastise himself to achieve a greater spirituality. As early as 1822, when he was but 17, he noted his ill health, seeing in it a reminder that he must improve his time and prepare himself for the future he had chosen. That show of determination in the face of illness was indicative of Emerson's steady pursuit of what throughout his lifetime he freely called "power." Power, in his Neoplatonist philosophy, was active spirit, or will, a form of dominion that an individual achieved by unlocking the informing spirit hidden in the material world. This state of active power, a dominion Emerson urged upon all who would listen, was attained when the individual joined his or her human history with natural history. At that point, he says in *Nature* (1836), the "currents of the Universal Being" circulate through him, and all dualities are fused into one (Whicher, 24). All dualities would, of course, include sickness and health, and inasmuch as this moment of unification amounts to a second birth in which the individual reenters the womb of nature to issue forth a new creation in spirit, an inherited disease (such as TB was thought to be) might have been sloughed off with the old material self. Here indeed was a triumph of spiritual power over the forces of necessity and fate. It was a triumph later formulated into a religion by another New Englander, Mary Baker Eddy, founder of Christian Science.

Though Emerson triumphed over his own tubercular demon, his first marriage, to Ellen Louisa Tucker in 1829, was doomed from the start by the disease, which ended her life a year and a half later. At her death her husband wrote that he was "strangely happy": "Her lungs shall no more be torn nor her head scalded by her blood nor her whole life suffer from the warfare between the force and delicacy of her soul and the weakness of her frame" (Rusk, 149). The reaction of her loved ones to Ellen Emerson's death echoed what would become the stock literary depiction of the death from tuberculosis of a young female. Only 19 when she died, her mother-in-law described her as "calm and undismayed at the approach of death—and in a prayerful and resigned state of mind committed herself and all her dear friends unto God— biding each of us around her Farewell" (Rusk, 149).

=   The Saintly Victim   =

Beth March in Louisa May Alcott's *Little Women* (1868–69) dies in just such a manner. The fictional March family is based on the family of Amos Bronson Alcott, Emerson's friend and disciple, and his daughter Louisa may have had Ellen Emerson in mind, as well as her own sister Elizabeth, when she wrote that Beth's illness made her appear "as if the mortal was being slowly refined away, and the immortal shining through the frail flesh with an indescribably pathetic beauty."[6] Though Elizabeth Alcott's death was long, hard, and full of a suffering that was eased only by opium, family accounts have it that at the end she was able to kiss her sisters and parents before falling into a peaceful sleep from which she did not waken. This New England style of consumptive death had also found its way into Harriet Beecher Stowe's *Uncle Tom's Cabin* (1852), where it is transported to the southern plantation of the St. Clares. Eva, the too-good-to-be-true little daughter of the slave owner St. Clare, is presented as a frail creature always dressed in white. The innocence symbolized by the color of her dress not only marks her off from the guilt associated with slavery but denotes the sickness to which she will succumb. When the illness comes it is not named, but we know from the author's description that the symptoms are those of tuberculosis. Night sweats make her long hair an unwelcome trial, and Eva requests that her curls be cut off so that she can give them to her friends before she dies. Calling to her bedside the household slaves and Uncle Tom, she presents each with a curl and her blessings. Toward the end of her illness she feels no pain, "only a tranquil, soft weakness, daily and almost insensibly increasing; and she was so beautiful, so loving, so trustful, so happy, that one could not resist the soothing influence of that air of innocence and peace which seemed to breathe around her."[7]

The cultic attitudes toward death and dying that developed in nineteenth-century America, so successfully satirized by Mark Twain in the figure of Emmeline Grangerford in *Huckleberry Finn* (1885), arose in large part from the tuberculosis mythos, which was reinforced by scenes such as these. When *Uncle Tom's Cabin* became the nation's most popular stage presentation, the death of little Eva was considered to be the height of pathos. Though antecedent to Alcott and Stowe, Edgar Allan Poe (who is said to have had tuberculosis) no doubt drew more heavily on the myth than he realized when he declared that the most universally affecting idea is the death of a beautiful woman. Poe would have had good reason to associate tuberculosis with the death of women, for his mother, his foster mother, and his wife all died of the disease.

= Henry David Thoreau =

Nothing could be further removed from this popular image of the dying child-woman, or from the parallel image of the consumptive poet, than the figure of Henry David Thoreau, Concord's rugged transcendentalist who died of the disease in 1862. The Walden pioneer was born into a family whose members were already marked by tuberculosis: both his father and paternal grandfather died of the disease, and it became apparent early in their lives that his two sisters and his brother were affected. Thoreau developed symptoms in 1836 while he was still at college, from which he temporarily withdrew. He recovered from the illness then, as he did from a number of subsequent attacks, a recovery rate that the fresh-air theory of treatment for pulmonary tuberculosis would attribute to his life spent largely out of doors.

Certainly his healthful way of life would have contributed to Thoreau's longevity—he died at 45—but even this could not prevent the disease from recurring at various intervals throughout his life. Thoreau's faithfully kept journal is silent about these occurrences, even the final one in 1861–62, and we learn of his suffering and of his attempts to regain his health from the letters and journals of others. His close friend Ellery Channing wrote of a ten-week spell of confinement in the winter of 1861, a long period of time for Thoreau to remain indoors, which must have caused him enormous distress. In a quasi-medical report on his friend's condition Channing comments on Thoreau's great weight loss, pulse rate of 56, coughing exacerbated by cold air, and "lack of respitory [sic] oxygenation."[8]

Of this enforced confinement and its cause we have one firsthand account, brief though it is, in a letter from Thoreau to his friend Daniel Ricketson written 22 March 1861. In it Thoreau says he is not yet looking for the return of spring, having not had any winter: "I took a severe cold about the 3 of Dec. which at length resulted in a kind of bronchitis, so that I have been confined to the house ever since. . . . Channing has looked after me faithfully—says he has made a study of my case, & knows me better than I know myself. . . . Of course, if I knew how it began, I should know better how it would end."[9] The indeterminate "it" in Thoreau's letter can as easily refer to the great questions of life as to his illness, and it is hard not to imagine him casting about in his mind to answer the riddle of a fate that seemed to have doomed him.

On the advice of his doctor, Thoreau tried the usual remedy of removal to a better climate. With typical nonconformity, he spurned the suggestions of the West Indies and southern Europe and chose instead the newly touted restorative virtues of Minnesotan air. The trip west provided him with an opportunity to see prairie gophers, Native Americans, and whole new botanical species dissimilar from those he had studied closely for years in New England. By midsummer it appeared that the trip had worked its magic and Thoreau returned home, but his biographer Walter Harding terms the western sojourn "a tragic failure" and points to the report of the *New York Tribune* for 26 July 1861 confirming Thoreau's poor health (Harding, 450).

The following winter, according to Harding, friends were describing Thoreau in terms of the classic symptoms: "[A] flush had come to his cheeks and an ominous brightness and beauty to his eyes, painful to behold. His conversation was unusually brilliant, and we listened with a charmed attention which perhaps stimulated him to continue talking until the weak voice could no longer articulate" (Harding, 455). Of his illness we have only this from Thoreau, in a letter to a young inquirer written two months before his death in 1862: "You ask particularly after my health. I *suppose* that I have not many months to live; but, of course, I know nothing about it. I may add that I am enjoying existence as much as ever, and regret nothing" (Harding, 457). The end came in May 1862; he is said to have had not the slightest struggle with death, only a gradual cessation of breathing. For those who know him best from the pages of *Walden*, it is difficult to imagine the gradual lessening of that voice—which rasps its convictions so compellingly in the first chapter—or the diminution of the breath of life that so wholly inspires the closing chapters and is perhaps best encapsulated in the exultant, "Walden was dead and is alive again."

= Walden =

The foreground of Thoreau's masterpiece includes illness and death sufficient to explain the despair that permeates the opening chapter of the book. In the winter of 1842 his brother John had contracted tetanus, a disease marked by rigidity of the jaws, seizures, and great pain, terminating quickly in death. There was no one in the world to whom Henry David was closer, and John's agonized 11-day dying was all but unbearable for his younger brother. Thoreau nursed John constantly and held him as he died. After the burial Thoreau went into a severe depression and then began to exhibit, with no physical cause, all the symptoms of tetanus. The symptoms were unfounded except in his mind, but they were a sign of just how closely Thoreau identified with his lost brother and friend.

Two weeks after John's death, Thoreau suffered another wrenching loss. Waldo Emerson, the five-year-old son of his friend and mentor, died of a childhood illness. A deep attachment had developed between Thoreau and the child when Thoreau lived with the Emerson family, and he mourned the loss greatly. It was probably because of the strength of the relationship between Thoreau and little Waldo that a year later Emerson recommended Thoreau as a tutor to his nephews, the sons of his brother William Emerson, whose family lived in Staten Island, New York. There was another reason, however, for the suggestion that Thoreau leave Concord for a time—his ill health. The tuberculosis had once again manifested itself, and as always, it was believed that a change of scene would be beneficial. Thoreau took the post eagerly, but illness, a pervading sense of loss, and an overwhelming homesickness combined to make him miserable during his entire stay. He lasted at the job only from May until November, returning home, as do so many homesick Americans, for Thanksgiving.

But even in Concord things did not go well for Thoreau. Though he proved successful in the family pencil manufacturing business, he was not interested in industry and left the factory operations to his father. In the spring of 1844 he suffered a most humiliating experience: he and a friend inadvertently set fire to a portion of the Concord woods while attempting to cook some freshly caught fish; the result was a considerable loss of property, which deeply angered the townspeople and caused them to refer to him for years after as a "woods-burner." To someone as appreciative of nature as Thoreau, it must have been particularly painful to be so castigated. In fact, the high value he placed on nature was an absolute, and his inability to attach a comparable worth to other aspects of life was one of his traits that put him so at odds with those around him. New Englanders worked hard on their land or at their jobs, but Thoreau saw in their labor only misspent time and, eventually, misspent lives. In the spring of 1845 he decided to declare his economic independence and take up residence for a time on the shores of Walden Pond, located a few miles outside of Concord, where he intended to prove his theory that, as we would say in modern parlance, less is more in this life. Two years of living close to nature were later compressed into one when, in *Walden* (1851), Thoreau described the practical application of transcendental principles in terms of a single year's natural cycle.

Every reader of *Walden* notes the progression in the work, from the materialism of a consumer society to the spiritualism of an existence built on the higher laws of nature. The economy rooted in the "necessaries of life" detailed at the beginning of the book is Thoreau's remedy for the economic ills not only of a postdepression America (he was witness to the severe effects of the 1837 depression) but of a society made ill by a consuming desire for material goods, for the "things" that Emerson claimed "ride mankind." While the transcendental philosophy inherent in this economy stretches back to touch an earlier Puritanism, it likewise reaches forward to impress its ideas on a later time. The pervasive aura of doubt and despair in late nineteenth-century America, identified by one cultural historian as antimodernism, had its antecedent in transcendentalist New England, among those more thoughtful, and spiritual, Americans of an earlier time.[10] Though Emerson and his fellow transcendentalists saw themselves firmly lodged within "the party of the future" and would have wondered at the medievalism and other more escapist manifestations of their turn-of-the-century successors, there was a link between early and late antimodernism.

The connection stemmed from a deep questioning of the industrial, capitalist economy and the harm it wrought to traditional values and to the spiritual life of the individual. In the first half of the century such questioning found an outlet in widespread experimentation with communal living, in which cooperation replaced competition, and in transcendentalist sanctification of nature and the individual self. Late in the century serious distrust of the relationship between capital and labor would give rise to the Marxian critique of capitalism, a quasi-medical approach that established causes, effects, and remedies for economic and social ills. Before Marx, however, one can detect in transcendentalist spirituality a distrust of the materialism spawned by industrialization, a dissent from the swelling tide of consumerism, and an uneasy sense that modern capitalism exhausted both man and nature. I am suggesting that for more spiritually inclined New Englanders of the first half of the century, such as Emerson and Thoreau, this materialism, this rampant consumerism, seemed to parallel the disease of tuberculosis, which first assumed epidemic proportions in New England, where industrialization began. (Later a similar but more focused connection was made: "neurasthenia," widely diagnosed among Americans at the turn of the century, was believed to result from attempts to keep up with the pace of modern life and maintain high economic standards, attempts that, it was believed, drained one's energy to the point of physical and psychological illness.)

The first chapter of *Walden*, "Economy," continues the jeremiad tradition of the New England Puritans: Thoreau warns against a spiritual declension, but from a new economic angle, in support of which he sets up an adversarial relationship between materialism and spiritualism. Only two years before taking up residence at Walden, while living in the Staten Island home of William Emerson, Thoreau had experienced—coincident with the recurrence of his tuberculosis—the emptiness of soul that can pervade a well-appointed house intended to bespeak its owner's affluence. Of the life of the Staten Island Emersons he wrote in his journal, "I have seen such a hollow, glazed life as on a painted floor. . . . The atmosphere of the apartments is not yet peopled with the spirits of its inhabitants; but the voices sound hollow and echo, and we see only the paint and the paper" (Harding, 155).

This intimate observation of a family life unlike that which he had known in New England, combined with the recurrence of his disease, leads Thoreau to insinuate into his later discussion of economy references to health as the perfect economy, or order, of the body. As he asserts in all his discussion of matter and spirit, this perfect economy is wholly dependent upon spirit. *Walden* contains numerous references to the sickness unto death of the spirit, an ailment that Thoreau associates with too great a care for the things of this world. The remedy is in all cases a certain relation to nature: "What is the pill which will keep us well, serene, contented? Not my or thy great-grandfather's, but our great-grandmother Nature's universal, vegetable, botanic medicines, by which she has kept herself young always" (*Walden*, 153). Similarly, his recurring references to material life and death are set against the immortality of spirit, as in the chapter. "Higher Laws." Here he speaks of the animal life of the body, which, he says, "may enjoy a certain health of its own; that we may be well, yet not pure" (*Walden*, 242). In describing the spiritual purity toward which we should aspire he approximates the stock image of the consumptive, whose body is etherealized and made perfect as the flesh falls away. "Yet the spirit," he tells us, "can for the time pervade and control every member and function of the body, and transmute what in form is the grossest sensuality into purity and devotion. . . . Man flows at once to God when the channel of purity is open. . . . He is blessed who is assured that the animal is dying out in him day by day, and the divine being established" (*Walden*, 243). In the chapter entitled "Spring" the return of natural life and the glory of early springtime light move him to the biblical affirmation of spirit and its immortality: "O Death, where was thy sting? O Grave, where was thy victory, then?" (*Walden*, 349).

In the concluding chapter of *Walden* Thoreau speaks of the advice given by doctors to consumptive patients (though he does not name the disease)— that they seek a change of scene and climate. He may have recalled to mind, as he wrote, the sickness of the body he experienced while living in Staten Island and the analogous sickness of soul he had observed among the more affluent in this world. Only then do we realize that in taking us into the woods at Walden, where we relive with him his excursion into the wilderness, Thoreau has reversed reality: rather than being the one who is ill, he has played the physician's role, removed us from our "sick" society, and led us on a journey toward spiritual health.

Thoreau's approach to the spiritual malady afflicting his society, though aggressive in tone, was much the same as that taken by medical science faced with the mystery of tuberculosis. Both conditions were spiritualized: the TB sufferer was perceived as becoming more and more ethereal as the disease progressed, just as, in Thoreau's economy, the materialist becomes more and more spiritually healthy as the disease of matter falls away. And what became the habit of American writers, omitting explicit reference to the disease, was aided by those habits of mind among nineteenth-century Americans that gave rise to a symbolic mode of thought and representation, rendering tuberculosis more tractable as symbol than as fact. The coincidence that brought tuberculosis to the foreground in America at the moment when an earlier allegorical mode of thinking was sliding into a more broadly sugges- tive symbolic mode established the metaphorical richness of the disease. All illness and disease lends itself to metaphor, since it is human to attempt to understand disease in a way that will justify our suffering. But to be sick in the land of the well is often to be suspect, and when a sickness spreads across the land, mysterious in its cause and cure, a people whose literary roots are largely biblical will build upon that base of spirituality and create correspond- ing images of the sickness.

Thoreau firmly locates the disease of materialism within society and posits the source of health in nature. He sees the sick soul as needing to remove itself from society and seek restoration in nature, because the illness is the result of a dysfunction not within the soul, but within the society. He goes even further and associates economic illness, which he claims afflicts so many of his fellow New Englanders, with the inheritance of debt-ridden properties:

> I see young men, my townsmen, whose misfortune it is to have inherited farms, houses, barns, cattle, and farming tools; for these are more easily acquired than got rid of. . . . They have got to live a man's life, pushing all these things before them, and get on as well as they can. How many a poor immortal soul have I met well-nigh crushed and smothered under its load, creeping down the road of life, pushing before it a barn, seventy-five feet by forty, its Augean stables

never cleansed, and one hundred acres of land, tillage, mowing, pasture, and wood-lot. The portionless, who struggle with no such unnecessary inherited encumbrances, find it labor enough to subdue and cultivate a few cubic feet of flesh. (*Walden*, 5–6)

Embedded in this passage is Thoreau's discontent with the breakup of the agricultural society based on family property ownership that had provided the social structure of New England before the Revolution. By the 1840s, when Thoreau was writing, some farmers had to work a farm for years to pay off its mortgage, and others who had inherited their land had to pay off its "encumbrances," or liens. The 100-acre inherited farms of which he speaks were but the remains of what had been large land holdings protected by entail and primogeniture. Though family owned, these large estates had been kept up and made productive by means of hired labor, the propertyless, who in Thoreau's time were commanding high wages in factories while other young men struggled to keep up their family farms. It is not property as such that Thoreau values, but the stability of the social order it provides and the emphasis in that order on each individual contributing his or her labor to a common good without being driven by the profit motive.

The cumulative effect of his enumeration of the things that weight the lives of these inheritors of the land makes all the more ponderous his end equation between the inherited land and the "few cubic feet of flesh" that even the portionless, despite their newfound prosperity, must carry. This flesh is their only inheritance, but it too must be subdued and cultivated to the ends of industry. The reference to the flesh also serves as a reminder that for many a New Englander the family inheritance included a history of tuberculosis. Thoreau seems to be drawing a corollary between poverty, of inheritors and portionless alike, and the prevailing illness—to which he makes no overt reference—when he says, "Some of you, we all know, are poor, find it hard to live, are sometimes, as it were, gasping for breath" (*Walden*, 7). The image, so evocative of the suffering of the tubercular, would not have gone unnoticed by contemporary readers.

The connection made between the image and the region's inherited land would not have gone unnoticed because in America, more so than in Europe, consumption had come to be accepted as a hereditary disease about which nothing could be done. As discussed in chapter 3, the environmental theory of disease prevailed in the eighteenth century, as a result of the preceding century's etiological view of illness. All the eighteenth-century discussions of climate and its effect on animal and human life in the New World grew out of the new emphasis on locating the source of illness outside the body, and out of the need to defend America from European-based attacks on the debilitating effects of nature in the New World. Early in the 1800s, however, when pulmonary tuberculosis appeared in succeeding generations of New Englanders, who had no understanding of its contagious nature and no use for the germ theory of infection, the disease was simply accepted as hereditary. Inevitably, some more analytical minds sought to understand the disease by connecting genealogy to environment. Theodore Parker (1810–60), the Unitarian minister who became transcendentalism's foremost orator (after Emerson), suffered with tuberculosis most of his adult life and died far from his beloved Boston, in Rome, where he had gone in hope of recovery. Unlike Thoreau, Parker showed a keen awareness of his disease, which he believed he had inherited from his mother, who had died of it. His journals and correspondence, especially his letters to his doctors, reveal a close attention to the symptoms and progress of the disease through years of ill health.

In one such letter, written to a Dr. Bowditch just two years before Parker's death, the minister provides his doctor with a detailed family history beginning with his first American ancestor, Thomas Parker, who left England in 1634 to settle in Massachusetts. As he traces his history through successive generations, Parker makes the point that there was "no consumption," but that in the third generation his forebear built "a great house." Parker provides all the details of the house's situation, including the condition of the adjacent land ("wet, springy, and spongy, with fogs often gathering"), the prevailing winds from which the house was spared by wooded hills, even the species of trees present in the nearby forests. No sign of consumption appeared in the next four generations of Parkers, all of whom lived in the family homestead, until the wife of a Parker died of TB, as did eight of his children and two grandchildren. One son of the diseased mother "moved from the family homestead, and settled on the piece of wet, spongy land, exposed to the bleakest west, north, and north-east wind"; all six of the children in this man's family died of consumption between the ages of 20 and 24.

From this history Parker draws for his physician the following inferences: "1) that the healthiest of families, living in such a situation as I have described, generation after generation, acquire the consumptive disposition, and so die thereof; 2) that it sometimes requires several generations to attain this result; 3) that members of the family born with this consumptive disposition often perish thereby, though they live and are even born in healthy localities."[11] The letter is a remarkably clear indication of the ways in which thoughtful Americans were attempting to understand how this "inherited" disease had entered their healthy family lines, and it provides insight into the theorizing that may have influenced Thoreau's thinking.

The feeling of helplessness in the face of a hereditary, mortal illness no doubt lies behind the desperate need to romanticize both the disease itself and those who were its victims. Indeed, the despairing note sounded early in *Walden*—"The mass of men lead lives of quiet desperation"—continues as a leitmotiv even into the "Conclusion," where Thoreau asks, "Why should we be in such desperate haste to succeed and in such desperate enterprises?" Throughout *Walden* Thoreau writes against this despair, countering its melancholy tread with his acute awareness of the rhythm of the natural world, and it is this spirit that leads him to the heroic statement, "If a man does not keep pace with his companions, perhaps it is because he hears a different drummer. Let him step to the music which he hears, however measured or far away. It is not important that he should mature as soon as an apple tree or an oak. Shall he turn his spring into summer?" (*Walden*, 358–59).

Surely one would not hasten the spring, or even the winter, of one's life if one was aware from childhood of the early death that was one's inheritance. Try though he might to rise on the wings of spiritual power above his own familial predisposition toward consumption, Emerson eventually bowed to it in 1860 as a part of the Fate that, in his essay, "Fate," he at last acknowledged as "the Beautiful Necessity": "How shall a man escape from his ancestors, or draw off from his veins the black drop which he drew from his father's or his mother's life? . . . His parentage determines it. Men are what their mothers made them" (Whicher, 334). This same sense of being what his mother made him, of the genetic heritage bequeathed to him in the womb, may have informed Thoreau's extraordinary letters to his mother during his stay on Staten Island, when he was once again in a tubercular condition. Only 25 years old and intolerably homesick, Thoreau uncharacteristically beseiged his family and friends in Concord with letters begging for news of home and wrote at length to his mother effusively thanking her for engendering in him by her lofty expectations whatever high degree of character he may have attained. "The thought of you will constantly elevate my life," he wrote, "it will be something always above the horizon to behold, as when I look up at the evening star" (Harding, 154). "Henry is very tolerant," was Mrs. Thoreau's restrained comment on these soulful letters, but they may have been Henry's attempt to absolve his mother of the part she had unwittingly played in dooming him to an early death. In a pre-Freudian world where hereditary disease was rampant, such a statement as Emerson's "Men are what their mothers made them" could be a terrible indictment.

Emerson never mentioned the cause of Henry David Thoreau's death in his moving tribute to his deceased friend, but he began and ended his eulogy with references to familial associations. At the outset he identifies Thoreau's French ancestry and speaks of him as the last male descendant of a family whose origins were in the Isle of Guernsey. In his concluding comments he says, "The country knows not yet, or in the least part, how great a son it has lost" (Whicher, 395). The expectancy that fueled the immigration of the thousands who had fled Europe and the ills of the Old World for the healthy promise of the New, is implied in these two references, as is the further, ironic thwarting of expectation in the dying out of the family name. Europe's writers found in tuberculosis a romantically charged subject (Thomas Mann's *The Magic Mountain* is a classic example), but in American writing there are only veiled references to the disease that cut short the promise of many a young life and many a family. Unnamed, it appears disguised in a metaphysical economy; it is the medical analogue of a philosophy rooted in the conviction that the remedy for a too highly valued materiality was an ever increasing spirituality. Seen in this light, *Walden* reflects its author's physical as well as spiritual condition as he gives public voice to what was in his time so personal a disease.

= The Sanitary Movement =

America's difficulty in publicly naming the disease of tuberculosis continued for a time even after the discovery of its cause, but in the post–Civil War years a new awareness that the spread of consumption was related to insufficient ventilation and poor sanitation began to permeate the American consciousness. In these same years the industrialization of American cities produced slums, crowded workshops, and more and more of the social ills that accompany mass urban enterprise. The new interpretation of tuberculosis as a product of this industrialization was something that Americans were prepared to accept, exposed as they were already to both the miasmic theory of disease—the belief that bad air caused disease—and the earlier romantic attachment to nature that had developed early in the century as part of a wave of nationalist feeling. Furthermore, Americans could cope with such an interpretation, for it offered the possibility of action: if TB was a disease of the city, the city dweller merely had to undertake a regimen of fresh air, good food, and walks in the park. Thanks to the parks movement, which started about midcentury, most major cities boasted green public recreation areas so that urbanites no longer had to resort to the use of cemeteries for exercise. Best of all, if tuberculosis was not a matter of inherited tendency, one could improve one's chances of escaping it by improving one's way of life. Here was something Americans could take hold of, and such groups as the Fresh Air Movement and The Outdoor Life swung into action.

When word came from Germany that Robert Koch had successfully cultured tubercle bacilli and had thus determined the bacterial nature of the disease, America was not impressed. Europe was on fire with excitement at the news, but in the United States, where medicine was still struggling to gain a hold in a society that had little patience for pure science, the discovery was treated with disinterest and even with some ridicule. This reaction was not solely attributable to a disdain for European pronouncements. Americans were just beginning to accept the notion that tuberculosis was a concomitant of poverty and unsanitary conditions and were hence unwilling to accept evidence that the disease originated in a contagious bacterium.

The environmentalist approach, unlike antimaterialistic transcendentalism, lent itself to a cause, even a crusade, in which corporate America could participate—the sanitary movement. Two of the outstanding corporations to take up the fight were Metropolitan Life Insurance Company, which mounted a huge educational program, and the Standard Oil Company of New Jersey, which entered the movement later. Corporate involvement seemed to be benevolent, but it was also opportunistic in that corporations were thus able to establish favorable alliances with government. Even more to the point, the sanitary movement contributed to the growing consolidation of power shared by corporate America and the medical profession.

The history of the medical profession in the post–Civil War years was one of increased professionalization, achieved by the formation of the American Medical Association (AMA), a restructuring of medical education, and a re-definition of medicine to deemphasize the idea of it as an art and shift the focus to the scientific research that had put European countries, such as France and Germany, so far ahead of America in medical knowledge. The AMA viewed political power as the key to this professionalization, and at the time political power was heavily vested in the capitalists whose huge corporations were making possible America's rise to the level of world power. Medicine improved its own condition by attaching itself to the power structure implicit in big business.[12] "Health is not merely analogous to capital, *it is capital*, the value of which to a certain extent may be expressed in coin," declared John Shaw Billings, one of the leading medical reformers of the late nineteenth century.[13] It was a sentiment that had the ring of truth about it to a people schooled in the Franklinian notion that "Time is money," and Billings's pronouncement that "Health is capital" sounds in the background of many a biography and literary work of the period, especially, as shall be seen, in the work of Henry James.

Under the influence of the sanitary movement, cleanliness became the watchword, and TB, no longer the disease of the educated and creative, became associated in the popular mind with the unwashed masses who appeared to create nothing but urban blight. Even when Koch's discovery eventually gained credence in America it was mainly as part of the effort to educate the public to the dangers of infection that accompanied a lack of careful sanitation. Children and young people, especially those living in large cities, were heavily targeted by the health crusaders—and with good reason, since they were extremely vulnerable to infection. Mark Caldwell's recent history of the battle waged in America against tuberculosis includes examples of the quasi-literary warnings produced for the youth of the nation that played upon their vulnerability by presenting them as victims of society. One such piece taught that,

> Mankind, not Death, is the stern foe of children
> It wins its gold through the toil of little fingers;
> Poisons the sweet blue air; lets fever burn
> From court to crowded court; taints meat and drink.[14]

In a neat shifting of responsibility away from the expanding monopolies of the time, which demanded "the toil of little fingers," a very generalized

"Mankind" is held responsible for the well-being of children, who are portrayed as sacrificial victims for economic gain by an abstract and impersonal power. In the story, the voice of Death calls the children away one by one until one child averts his destiny by joining the National Tuberculosis Association.

The voices of the progressive reformers calling the American public to take collective responsibility for the evils wrought by an industrial rapaciousness were in fact misdirected, for given the alliances between corporate industry and politics—and the pressure exerted within a capitalist economy for ever greater profits—the needed reforms were not within the immediate power of the public to effect. At the beginning of the twentieth century the progressive movement was able to tighten the leash on corporate power, but in the earlier absence of such reformist activities Americans had been forced to depend upon the philanthropies of such masters of capitalism as John D. Rockefeller and Andrew Carnegie. In his 1889 *North American Review* essay, "Wealth," Carnegie spells out a hierarchy of values different from the spirit-over-matter values of the transcendentalists and more in line with the social Darwinism of the time. The accumulation of wealth by some is "inevitable" under capitalism's law of competition, he claims, and society should welcome the resultant inequality as a sign that the best are rising to positions of control. The responsibility, however, of administering this wealth was great; Carnegie believed that accumulated profits should not be left to one's heirs but should be placed in trust for the good of as many as possible. Carnegie followed his own recommendations for the use of wealth: giving to universities and medical schools, establishing libraries, supporting public parks, and providing concert halls. It was not long before the essay had been dubbed the "Gospel of Wealth," and though some excoriated him (especially the clergy, since Carnegie gave little money to religious institutions), most people in America subscribed to his ideas and were grateful for his benefactions.

= "Paul's Case" =

Willa Cather lived in Pittsburgh for ten years, working as a reporter for a city newspaper and as a city employee. From there she went to New York to join the staff of *McClure's*, the notorious muckraking magazine and tool of the progressive movement. Cather had become very familiar with Pittsburgh and its Carnegie steel factories, its smoke-filled air, and its grubby working-class neighborhoods. She understood how hard it could be for a young person who simply did not fit into the workday atmosphere of such a city, and who might develop a hunger for the glamour of the world of art brought into view by the philanthropy of an Andrew Carnegie. But Cather's own understanding of art was that it demanded of both artist and audience the highest moral and spiritual integrity, and that it must not be profaned by mass secularization or the trappings of a cheap glamour.

Although Carnegie was not a principal target of *McClure's*, which aimed most of its ire at Rockefeller's Standard Oil, all of the captains of industry were fair game as the magazine's writers sought out the tenuous but significant connections between the nation's economic interests and its political power. In 1905 Samuel Hopkins Adams produced a series of articles for *McClure's* in which he examined the conditions of tenement life; he found there everything that made possible the spread of contagious diseases, best exemplified by the scourge of tuberculosis. In the same year *McClure's* published Cather's "Paul's Case," one of the finest examples of the magazine's pioneering efforts at bringing realistic fiction into periodicals. To my knowledge, "Paul's Case" has never been viewed in light of either the national tuberculosis awareness campaign or of Carnegie's Gospel of Wealth, but it hints strongly at both.

In recent years "Paul's Case" has become one of the most frequently anthologized of Willa Cather's short stories. It deserves this attention, for it is not only a first-rate work but an excellent example of Cather's economy of language: every word counts toward the cumulative effect of the story, including the title. Precisely what is meant by Paul's "case"? Only once in the story is it mentioned directly, when the members of a theatrical stock company, amused by Paul's extravagant stories about his associations with them, agree with the faculty of Paul's high school and with his father, "that Paul's was a bad case."[15] *Stagestruck* might be the word to describe Paul's condition, but the emphasis given the word *case* by its use in the title suggests something more than the kind of adolescent fancy that fastens on the theater world.

Cather subtitled the story "A Study in Temperament"; her subject is a high-school boy who is "something of the dandy" in dress and manner. His favorite accessory is a red carnation in his buttonhole, which sets him off from his contemporaries and, in fact, from most others in his Pittsburgh neighborhood. Paul lives with his father and sisters on Cordelia Street, a place where people sit on the front stoop and tally up their days and lives in terms of how many items they turned out in the factory and how many waffles were eaten at the church supper. Looming above them all are the smokestacks of the steel-producing plant that darkens with grime the houses, streets, and people, who are all in some way dependent upon it. The name of the steel company is never mentioned, but Paul works as an usher in Carnegie Hall, which serves to identify it as part of the Carnegie beneficence that accompanied the creation of the Pittsburgh steel-making empire.

Only at Carnegie Hall does Paul really come alive. There he can lose himself in the paintings in the picture gallery or in the sights and sounds of concert performers and their audiences. "It was not that symphonies, as such, meant anything in particular to Paul," Cather is careful to explain, "but the first sigh of the instruments seemed to free some hilarious and potent spirit within him; something that struggled there like the Genius in the bottle found by the Arab fisherman. He felt a sudden zest of life" ("Case," 246). The bottled-up spirit that, once freed, reveals its potency with a sudden zest not *for* life but *of* life is symbolized by the red carnation Paul wears, a symbol that in turn signifies the sanguinary temperament for which Paul's "case" provides a study. Cather is using temperament here in its medieval application—to the four aqueous humors that govern the health of the body, blood, phlegm, and bile, yellow and black. The red carnation signifies the prevailing humor, blood, governing Paul's temperament and suggests, as well, the tell-tale sign of blood, with which the consumptive's cough is associated.

Paul himself is a figure in stark contrast to this temperamental suggestion of blood-zest. Tall and "very thin, with high, cramped shoulders and a narrow chest," the boy has eyes "remarkable for a certain hysterical brilliancy" and "a glassy glitter about them" ("Case," 243). He wears a set smile but is "always glancing about him, seeming to feel that people might be watching him and trying to detect something" ("Case," 244). What he is trying to conceal is hinted at by one of his teachers, who feels there is "something sort of haunted" about Paul's smile and explains, "The boy is not strong, for one thing. I happen to know that he was born in Colorado, only a few months before his mother died out there of a long illness. There is something wrong about the fellow" ("Case," 245). The "something wrong" is never defined beyond the narrator's judgmental offering that Paul has no desire to be a musician, an actor, an artist, or any of the vocations for which he has such an insatiable craving: "He felt no necessity to do any of these things; what he wanted was to see, to be in the atmosphere, float on the wave of it, to be carried out, blue league after blue league, away from everything" ("Case," 252).

Forced to leave school and go to work, denied access to the theater and the concert hall, Paul steals money from his employer and leaves Pittsburgh for a fling in New York City. When he reflects on his thievery it is with a sense of relief, for he feels that he has at last thrown down the gauntlet to "the thing in the corner" that all his life "seemed always to be watching him" ("Case," 255). After a week of enjoying all that Manhattan has to offer, he learns from a newspaper story that the theft has been repaid by his father and that the firm will not prosecute; instead, his father is on his way to the eastern city, where his son has been seen, with the intention of returning him to home and Sunday School. Prison would have been preferable, Paul feels, and with an absolute calm he goes about what must be done. He is not at all afraid, "perhaps because he had looked into the dark corner at last and knew. It was bad enough, what he saw there, but somehow not so bad as his long fear of it had been" ("Case," 259–60).

A short train ride to Newark, New Jersey, and a cab drive following the tracks out of town brings Paul to his destination. Once in the country he leaves the cab and walks through heavy, drifted snow to a small hill beneath which run the railroad tracks. He notices that the red carnation on his coat is drooping from the cold, and he thinks of how flowers, "in spite of their brave mockery at the winter," have "only one splendid breath," and that "it was a losing game in the end" ("Case," 260). He takes the carnation from his coat, makes a hole in the snow, and buries the fading blossom. When a train approaches on the tracks below, he jumps. He feels "something strike his chest," and his body is thrown into the air.

To read this story in the context of the history of tuberculosis in America is to recognize something of the country's changing perceptions of the disease and the way in which American writers have chosen to mask it in metaphor. From the physical description of the boy, one can conclude that Paul's is the case history of a child born to a woman who was already dying of tuberculosis and who had been drawn to the dry air of Colorado in a futile search for health. His siblings show no signs of the disease, but Cather is nonetheless writing within the framework of the earlier belief in TB as an inherited disease. The red carnation Paul wears in his buttonhole suggests the bloodied sputum of the tubercular (as well as the traditional associations with passion and eroticism), but in Cather's study of temperament it also suggests the fevered blood that dominates Paul's physical being and determines his personality. The author builds upon the earlier concept of the tubercular personality as one exhibiting extremes of youthfulness, sensitivity, and creativity but departs from it by making Paul into a lover of glamour rather than of art. His desire to float on the wave of art and be carried away by it is symptomatic of the superficial appreciation of the arts that is the most he can hope to attain. When he attempts to inflate his shallow adoration into something more, he can do so only by stealth: he purloins, as it were, the objects of his romantic fascination by stealing the means to obtain them. Worst of all, for Paul, his theft forces him to come to terms with the knowledge that has always lurked in the dark corner of his mind, the awareness of how brief and showy, like the "brave mockery" of a flower in winter, his life will be, and how his stolen pleasure will expire after "only one splendid breath."

"Paul's Case" is a bitter story for a number of reasons, not the least of which is its author's conviction, firmly held throughout her life, that art is a high and holy creed demanding the purest of followers. After its initial appearance in *McClure's*, the story was included in a 1905 collection of Cather's stories, each of which deals with art in conflict with the mundaneness of American life. Entitled *The Troll Garden*, the book's epigraph was this stanza from Christina Rossetti's "Goblin Market" (1862), with its implication of contagion and contamination:

> We must not look at Goblin men,
> We must not buy their fruits:
> Who knows upon what soil they fed
> Their hungry thirsty roots?[16]

Paul hungers and thirsts for a more glamorous, if not a better life than that of his father and his neighbors, but it is not specifically his greediness that Cather warns against. To allude to tuberculosis without naming it, and to make it a metaphor for the fevered shallowness of Paul's appreciation for the arts, is to suggest another form of consumption in a way that is similar to, though far more subtle than Thoreau's denunciation of economic excess. Cather was an elitist when it came to art and its true appreciation, and as her writing attests, she did not hesitate to protest its debasement. The frequent use in this story of the Carnegie name, the references to the dominating steel mill, and the fact that it is a railroad train, the source of so much of Carnegie's wealth, that ends Paul's life, all hint at the avarice of the "Robber Baron" and his feverish consumption of art as if it were a commodity to be bought—or if need be, stolen—and distributed as largesse, in the manner Carnegie had recommended in his Gospel of Wealth. The infectiousness of such a notion, evident in the ready acceptance of Carnegie's ideas, is revealed in the ease with which Paul succumbs to it. Cather can be said to have joined, in her own way, the national antituberculosis cause with the publication of this story, though the danger to American youth it suggests is consumption of quite another kind, the "consumption" of art as commodity. Nonetheless, "Paul's Case" continues the use, begun in the preceding century, of tuberculosis as a disease metaphorically representative of the ravages wrought by rampant materialism.

= The Sanatorium: In the Familial Mode =

In addition to the national crusade against tuberculosis, which was waged largely in the cities, a second response to the disease swept this country as it did Europe: the belief in the curative effect of the sanatorium, of the type made famous in Thomas Mann's *The Magic Mountain*. (New York's world-renowned facility at Saranac Lake was the site of the highly publicized convalescence of the British writer Robert Louis Stevenson.) Though the word *sanatorium* was carefully chosen to denote the healing intent (from *sanare*, to heal), the sanatorium was in a sense an outgrowth of the idea of sanitation as a preventative measure against TB: clean air, clean beds, clean bodies, clean everything. The sanatorium was designed, however, for the treatment of those who had already contracted the disease. Typically, they were built in mountainous regions or near lakes, and they employed a regimen of enforced rest, wholesome food, and exposure to fresh air. A sanatorium was a place ruled by a high sense of purpose and principle, and the patient was expected to cooperate fully in his or her own recovery. Instilling this sense of shared responsibility required supervisory methods that to this point had been associated with prisons, and that return us to the earlier notion of medical power arrived at through surveillance.

The sanatorium movement began in the United States about 1875, though in Europe its origins reached back some three decades earlier. In constructing the necessary facilities, the cellular model offered by the penitentiary was transformed into an arrangement in which a simulated family of a small number of patients (of the same sex) lived in cottages set out on a large piece of land. Central to all the cottages was an administration building from which issued rules and regulations covering the minutest details of patients' daily lives as well as the measures designed to enforce them. Patients were regularly reminded that they were engaged, jointly with the administrators of the sanatorium, in warfare against the disease. Discipline was required, as in any army, and infractions of rules looked upon as a dereliction of duty, not so much to one's self but to American society in general.

The financial sponsorship of the sanatoriums was drawn from many sectors—government, private enterprise, voluntary associations, and the medical profession—reinforcing the notion of societal responsibility. Great sums of money were needed to build and maintain the sanatoriums, and since every segment of society was affected by tuberculosis, every segment was called upon to do its part. Many Americans will recall the Christmas Seals bearing the emblem of the National Tuberculosis Association—thousands of which were sold annually to raise money for the cure and treatment of TB— and the collections taken up in movie theaters for regional sanatoriums. In this we see evidence of the kind of centralized governmental control of medicine that developed in eighteenth-century France diffusing into what in America becomes the interlocking interests of medicine, politics, and business. Because tuberculosis had not initially been understood as contagious, it had not received the same kind of governmental attention as had other clearly epidemical diseases, such as yellow fever and cholera. Hence no public regulatory agency took charge, not even to enforce the sanitary measures that were widely instituted at the end of the nineteenth century. The antituberculosis movement remained largely an association of big businesses and voluntary groups working with the medical profession and government. Although all segments of society benefited from the movement, the medical community emerged from it a much more powerful entity than it had been.

The measure of this increased power might be said to have been symbolized by the profession's primary method of treatment, the sanatorium, which by its confinement and supervision of patients reenacted historically valid attempts to separate and regulate those who presented a threat to society. As is usual in institutional construction, architectural design implemented the supervisory role of the sanatorium, even providing, by its cottage format, the suggestion of a community based on society's basic unit, the family. Interestingly, it was the family that had most come under attack earlier in the century from economic reformers advocating socialism.

Fundamental to the socialist attack on the system of free enterprise and on the concept of individualism as it had developed in Jacksonian America was the belief that the family was the place where a destructive sense of competition was bred. The communitarian societies and associative groups that sprang up across America during the reform years, 1820–1860, aimed, in one way or another, at reforming the idea of the traditional family. Whether by explicit reeducation of its members or by implicit doctrinal teachings that contradicted familial attachments, the object was the same—the obliteration of what had been accepted as the "natural" family order. What these communities offered in its place was a new type of group relationship in which all the members functioned as an extended family but none was allowed to develop proprietary feelings toward any others in the group.

That American families were faltering and in need of help seems to be evident from the creation in midcentury of children's reformatories in numerous states and from the large numbers of children who were given over to the Society of Shakers to be raised in their communities. (The most successful of the communitarian groups, the Shakers were forbidden to marry. Dependent upon conversions for their continuation, they welcomed children into their midst as potential converts.) Unlike the celibate Shakers, however, the state-operated reformatories supported the idea of the family but imposed upon its charges a supervision deemed lacking in their original families. In principle, then, the role of the reformatory was to take over the familial responsibility without abandoning the idea of the family as the ideal formative agent in society (Rothman, 234). The obvious support for the traditional idea of the family was expressed in the design of the reformatories, which—like the TB sanatoriums—followed a cottage plan that provided for supervisory personnel.

This belief in the sanctity of the family permeated American society in the nineteenth century, but as the century wore on it became more and more difficult for families to function according to the ideal. Even before the advent of the multitudinous social ills readily encountered in the post–Civil War industrial cities, poverty and alcoholism were frequent causes of dysfunctional families. By the middle of the century alcoholism was one of the nation's most serious social problems because from it stemmed so many other ills that affected the order of both family and society, including chronic unemployment and domestic violence. Despite the extent of the problems facing families, the family as an institution remained so idealized that the sanatorium movement endorsed the family structure almost unanimously in choosing not only designs for its facilities but treatments for TB sufferers. Whether or not the treatment of tuberculosis was facilitated by maintaining the semblance of a functioning family remains an unproven theory; but the theory is bolstered by the only instance in American literary history of a well-known author who was a patient in such an institution writing about the experience.

= Eugene O'Neill =

Tuberculosis did not enter American literature directly—that is, it was not identified by name—until the twentieth century when the playwright Eugene

O'Neill first broached the subject. O'Neill was a highly autobiographical writer, and it is no wonder that so dramatic an event as his contracting tuberculosis while a young man would find its way into his plays. Three of O'Neill's plays tell the story in one way or another—*Beyond the Horizon* (1920), *The Straw* (1919), and *Long Day's Journey into Night* (1956)—and in each the topic is interwoven with the theme of family.

O'Neill became ill in the autumn of 1912, when he was 24. At the time he was working as a reporter for the *New London Telegraph* and living with his family at what was referred to then as a summer cottage, though it was a large old Connecticut house. Convinced at first that he had nothing more than a persistent summer cold, O'Neill soon found it hard to ignore both his persistent symptoms of a graver illness and his mother's frightened retreat into her morphine addiction. Ella O'Neill's father had died of TB, and she was morbidly fearful of losing her son (whose difficult birth had started her on the path of addiction to the pain-relieving substance) to the same illness. By November the diagnosis had been made, and a nurse was brought into the household to attend young Eugene. After a month he had not improved, only gradually worsened, and the decision was made to hospitalize him. Here is where Eugene and his father, a touring stage actor of some success but a man known for his frugality, came into open conflict. James O'Neill insisted that his son enter the state-run charity sanatorium in Fairfield County. Eugene and his father fought over this, and though the son did his father's bidding, he remained at the sanatorium for only two days, after which he left for New York City. At this the father became fearful for his son's recovery and had him admitted to the privately run Gaylord Farm Sanatorium in Wallingford, Connecticut.

Gaylord was operated by Dr. David Lyman, one of the founders of the National Tuberculosis Association. As might be expected, the sanatorium was one of the best in the country and followed the cottage plan. By O'Neill's own testimony, it was at Gaylord that he first had the chance to sort out and assimilate his experiences and begin to put them into words.[17] Though romantic encounters between the patients at Gaylord were forbidden, Eugene had a brief fling with a young Irish girl and also made many friends within the family atmosphere that prevailed there. He became especially close to Dr. Lyman, and one suspects that the doctor filled in the young man's life the father role to which James O'Neill was unsuited. Eugene's stay was limited to six months, but he continued to write to the doctor for years and in one letter confessed that the recollections of his stay "are, and always will be, among the most pleasant of my memories" (Gelb, 238).

His experience at the Gaylord Farm Sanatorium furnished material for one of O'Neill's earliest plays, *The Straw*. Written in the realistic style of his early period, the play provides the sole literary picture we have of a tuberculosis patient undergoing the enforced rest that offered his only hope of a cure. Rest meant not becoming emotionally involved, but Stephen Murray, who is

O'Neill's counterpart, instigates a romance with a young Irish working girl, Eileen Carmody. Stephen gains from the romance—even gaining weight—while Eileen loses. The scene in which the patients line up to be weighed and some reveal their anguish over a pound lost is a poignant depiction of what was a common occurrence. Stephen is soon well enough to leave and is surprised to learn that Eileen has taken their romance seriously. Left without him she becomes dangerously ill, but Stephen returns with an offer of marriage and a promise of removal to the West, where he believes she will get well. The play ends with an emphasis on Stephen's optimism, "the straw" of hope to which a drowning man will cling.

The Straw is particularly interesting for the contrast it establishes between Eileen Carmody's family and the community of patients, doctors, and nurses who together create a kind of "family" much closer to the ideal. The contrast is presaged in the first-act scene in the Carmody home where we meet Eileen. Although ill, she must take care of her four siblings, her responsibility since the death of their mother a year ago. The father is a drunkard who does not provide well for his family, bullies his children, and complains of the cost of Eileen's medicine. When the doctor arrives and tells him that Eileen must enter a sanatorium, Carmody says he cannot spare her from the family; only the doctor's threat to report him to the Tuberculosis Society has an effect on this sorry excuse for a father.

In contrast to the dismal Carmody family is the kinship demonstrated in a later scene in the main building of the sanatorium where the patients will soon gather for the weekly weighing in. As Dr. Stanton, director of the facility, talks with his staff he is revealed to be a kind, fatherly man who shows sympathy and understanding and who seems to be the inspiration for the hopefulness with which the play concludes. The dissimilarity between the doctor and Eileen's father is heightened when Carmody arrives at the sanatorium, loudly and abusively drunk. The family feeling exhibited among the patients and those who care for them extends to the final scene, when we sense that Stephen's feeling for Eileen, perhaps tempered by her illness, is really the affection of a sympathetic and caring brother more than the passion of a lover.

In the year he wrote The Straw O'Neill wrote another play in which the main character has tuberculosis, but in Beyond the Horizon (a Pulitzer Prize winner in 1921) the disease serves mainly to point up the general failure of Robert Mayo's life. The play expounds the double loss when neither of two brothers in a family lives his life according to his own wishes.

The culmination of O'Neill's attempts to deal with the tuberculosis episode in his life is Long Day's Journey into Night, considered by many to be his masterpiece. Written between 1939 and 1941, the play tells the story of the Tyrone family: the actor father, James; the morphine-addicted mother, Mary; a son, Jamie, who is an alcoholic wastrel; and his younger brother, Edmund, a cub reporter for a local newspaper. The time is the summer of

1912, and the place a cottage located in a Connecticut town. The father and his elder son have little regard for one another, the mother is lost in a fog of memories and addiction, and the younger son is ill and displaying symptoms of the disease that killed his mother's father. In the course of the play James Tyrone discusses with Edmund the state farm where he intends to send him for the tuberculosis cure, but when Edmund objects James relents and agrees to send him instead to a private institution. The play centers on the mother, on her lost state and her lost religious faith, but mostly on her denial of what she has become. In the final scene she wanders about in a drugged stupor reliving an earlier, happier time in her life, all unaware of the physical presence of her husband and sons. When Edmund rushes to her and tries to get her to acknowledge him by crying out, like a child, "I've got consumption," she rejects him, preferring to remain within her dream world. The play ends with father and sons standing immobile, staring at the wife and mother who treasures them in memory but cannot cope with present reality.

All the major elements of O'Neill's family life are represented in the play. It does not depict so dispirited a family as the Carmodys in *The Straw*, but the Tyrone-O'Neill family was clearly not the family the author would have liked it to be. That this, O'Neill's greatest work and the one in which he struggles to come to terms with his family, is set in the summer when he contracted tuberculosis reveals the emotional impact of that event on his life. Strangely, the father in the play comes off better than one might expect, chiefly by respecting his son's wish not to be sent to the charity farm and rescinding his original decision to do so. Perhaps O'Neill found it in his heart to forgive his own father and, in writing the play, may have been able to make peace with him as a result of having formed the surrogate-father relationship with Dr. Lyman. No similar relationship existed to exonerate his mother, evidently, for there is no forgiveness in this play for Ella O'Neill, not even a recognition that she did manage to overcome her addiction. By deliberately withholding this mark of her courage, O'Neill relegates her to a position of continued disease and dependency, while he rises above his illness. O'Neill may even have harbored some feelings of resentment toward his mother out of a belief that he had inherited the tubercular tendency from her family. Obviously he held her responsible for the failure of their family to live up to the ideal, dictated by American society, of what a family should be; none of the mothers in O'Neill's plays, unless they are dead, fares well in the playwright's hands. It may be that O'Neill had looked to his mother for a kind of centralized authority that she was unable to provide, thus leaving the family without the structure he felt it needed. In contrast, the family of patients and staff at the sanatorium had this structure because of the order imposed on it, first by the illness, which served to curb individual freedom, and then by the rules that regulated the congregate life in the cottages.

Historical circumstances have required of the American family a strength that it has not always been able to muster; perhaps as a reflection of this, our literature lacks examples of strong, formative families. (One thinks of the childhood classics, among which *Little Women* stands out for its picture of family life; but it is a family from which the father is noticeably absent.) Given the need for collective family strength in any society, but particularly in a frontier democracy, the position of a sick family member is roughly equivalent to that of the sick person in a democratic society, as described by the American sociologist Talcott Parsons. Parsons claims that the legitimation of the role of the sick individual in a democracy is dependent upon that individual's motivation toward health. Since sickness is viewed in America as a deviation from the norm of health, it is necessary for the sick person to acknowledge his or her deviancy and cooperate in the recovery of health.[18] The family-society has a responsibility to seek out or provide the necessary means of recovery, but it is the obligation of the sick person to "work at" getting well; when there is no evidence of this "work," the individual's motives become suspect, and the fear of contagion—of being infected not with the illness but with the sick person's lack of proper motivation—sets in. Parsons overtly connects illness with other types of deviance such as crime "and the breakdown of commitment to the values of the society," including moral values.

The contagion of indolence is the twentieth-century equivalent of the contagion of sin in Puritan New England and of the contagion of poverty and crime to nineteenth-century social reformers. Just as the nineteenth-century penitentiary inmate had a responsibility to absorb the work ethic, the sick of our time are perceived as having a responsibility to society to cooperate in getting well. Eugene O'Neill demonstrates his awareness of this responsibility by making the main character in *Beyond the Horizon*, the brother who is the greatest failure in a generally unsuccessful family, an unrecoverable tubercular. In *Long Day's Journey* he absolves himself of his own illness and displaces his anxiety at having been the one to fall victim to it by casting his mother in the role of the unrecoverable. It is she, not he, whose failure is made the centerpiece of the final scene: the other family members fall silent and gaze on her, spectators of her moral dissolution.

= The Wings of the Dove =

By far the most extraordinary use of tuberculosis by an American writer appears in Henry James's *The Wings of the Dove*, in which the metaphoric interchange of disease and money drives the plot. In large part this interchange reflects a trend in James's work toward greater use of monetary images in the fictive exploration of the exercise of power.[19] It also suggests James's acceptance of the idea referred to earlier, that the widespread appearance of tuberculosis in America was to some a sign of the human enervation that inevitably accompanied the nation's industrial economy, and to others, especially in New England, the sign of a contest between matter and spirit.

James could hardly have failed to note the increasing power of the medical profession in his native country; his own brother, William, had been a physician before entering the new field of psychology. And for reasons that will soon be made clear, the dictum of the medical reformer John Shaw Billings, "Health is capital," is not likely to have escaped James. Ultimately, the most interesting feature of James's use of money in conjunction with tuberculosis in *The Wings of the Dove* is its reflection of another form of economy, one that links health and wealth to the power to shape the lives of others.

The Wings of the Dove is the last major American literary work to in any way allude to the subject of tuberculosis. Written in 1902, the book belongs to James's "major phase," that is, to the final stage of his long career as a novelist and writer of short stories. But the term refers to more than mere chronology or periodicity; it signifies his achievement of a mastery of the art of writing fiction that few others have reached. At this point in his career James exhibits complete freedom in his art, by which he allows his imagination to shape and develop every idea and every word, drawing from each the fullest possible meaning. In these final works his sentences are long and convoluted, finely spun webs that mirror the intricate action of the plots they describe. As William Dean Howells facetiously pointed out, there are a great many words in these Jamesian masterpieces. Howells's "complaint" can only bring to mind the possibly apocryphal anecdote of a similar quibble raised by Mozart's royal patron, that the composer had employed too many notes in writing one of his operas. That kind of Mozartean artistic profligacy, apparent in James's final works, is the economic basis upon which the present study of *Wings* will ultimately rest.

The determining factor in the development of James's final stage, during which he wrote four novels, was the author's conscious decision to abandon plans to serialize his work in literary magazines. (*The Ambassadors* was actually completed before *Wings* but appeared in book form after it in 1903, because of a prior commitment to serialize the work in the *North American Review*.) Immediately, then, *The Wings of the Dove*, the novel in which James's heroine is dying of tuberculosis, fell under the influence of a new kind of literary economy: it would not bring its author the surety of payment that serialization promised, but released from the spatial constraints imposed by that medium, the author was free to invest as much of his art as he wished in its creation.

James chose to invest this economic and artistic freedom in a story he had long wanted to tell, though for the time its subject matter was questionable. As he says in the preface to the 1909 New York Edition, "[T]here are subjects and subjects, and this one seemed particularly to bristle."[20] The subject, of dubious propriety, "involved, to begin with, the placing in the strongest light a person infirm and ill—a case sure to prove difficult and to require much handling." (*Wings*, vi). James was conscious of the disgust and repulsion that disease aroused in the minds of many but nevertheless endowed his heroine with great wealth as well as disease. The combination is not surprising for, as we shall see, the idea of health as something that could be invested or even wasted had an uncommon hold on James's thinking.

The Wings of the Dove is one of James's explorations of the international theme, of the behavior of Americans abroad. Within that thematic frame are his stories of the American "girl" encountering European mores, *Daisy Miller*, *The Portrait of a Lady* (1881), *The Golden Bowl* (1904), and *The Wings of the Dove*. The heroine of *Wings* is Milly Theale, a young American woman who is the last surviving member of a prominent New York family, described as a "luxuriant tribe . . . of free-living ancestors" (*Wings*, 111) from whom Milly has inherited extraordinary wealth. From the point at which her illness is revealed—she suffers from a disease that, though unnamed, is symptomatic of tuberculosis—the connection between the disease and the victim's economic status is implied. Her hinted-at tuberculosis appears even to be part of Milly's weighty inheritance: James refers to her wealth as "the mass of money so piled on the girl's back" (*Wings*, 106). Despite this, she is "a young person with the world before her" (a deliberate echoing of Milton's *Paradise Lost*), a "princess," in the eyes of her New England friend, Susan Stringham, and "the potential heiress of all the ages" (*Wings*, 109).

Advised by her doctor to seek a change of scene, Milly heads for Europe with Mrs. Stringham, who is a writer of short stories for "the best magazines" (an interesting grace note from James, who had so recently renounced the role). Our first real view of Milly comes through the eyes of her companion, an older woman who is much concerned for the heiress's well-being. In establishing the relationship between the two women James heavily underscores Mrs. Stringham's powers of observation: "[F]or Mrs. Stringham, when she saw anything at all, saw much, saw everything" (*Wings*, 104); and, "Susan privately settled it that Boston was not in the least seeing [Milly]. . . . *She* was seeing her" (*Wings*, 105). These powers of observation are brought fully to bear upon their primary object when Susan Stringham searches for Milly, who has struck out on her own to follow a path in the Swiss Alps, comes upon the girl, and stops to gaze on her, unseen. Susan feels her attention to be "secretive," but her observation "scientific." "She struck herself as hovering like a spy, applying tests, laying traps, concealing signs" (*Wings*, 117). As she gazes on Milly—using her "scientific" mode of observation—Mrs. Stringham contemplates the young woman's princesslike quality, which she fancies to be a weight upon her companion's head, and concludes that this quality that so makes the difference between Milly and herself is all the result of having money. "[O]ur observant lady," James says, "had by this time repeatedly reflected that if one were talking of the 'difference,' it was just this, this incomparably and nothing else, that when all was said and done most made it" (*Wings*, 121). Though, to her friend's eyes, Milly is the least vulgar person one could imagine, everything about her reveals the quality her money is able to purchase: "She couldn't have lost it if she had tried—

that was what it was to be really rich. It had to be *the* thing you were," Mrs. Stringham comments privately (*Wings*, 121).

Susan's covert observation of Milly Theale concludes on a potentially frightening note when she sees Milly sitting on the edge of a precipice. The impression made on Mrs. Stringham is that the girl is lost in meditation: "She was looking down on the kingdoms of the earth, and though indeed that of itself might well go to the brain, it wouldn't be with a view of renouncing them. Was she choosing among them or did she want them all?" (*Wings*, 124). The question of "allness" and of Milly's determination, as her companion understands it, to take "full in the face the whole assault of life" (*Wings*, 125), comes to the fore in the first conversation between the two women to which we are privy. Milly has raised the subject of her illness, the exact nature of which remains a mystery to her, in an effort to learn if her doctor has imparted some knowledge of it to Mrs. Stringham. Her companion expresses concern:

> "Are you in trouble—in pain?"
> "Not the least bit. But I sometimes wonder—!"
> "Yes"—she pressed: "wonder what?"
> "Well, if I shall have much of it."
> Mrs. Stringham stared. "Much of what? Not of pain?"
> "Of everything. Of everything I have."
> . . . "You 'have' everything; so that when you say "much" of it—"
> "I only mean," the girl broke in, "shall I have it for long? That is
> if I *have* got it."
> . . . "If you've got an ailment?"
> "If I've got everything," Milly laughed.
> "Ah *that*—like almost nobody else."
> "Then for how long?" (*Wings*, 130–31)

This entire exchange is quoted to point up its deliberate ambiguity, which leaves the reader uncertain as to precisely what is being spoken of, whether pain, disease—and specifically, the disease of tuberculosis—or money. The only certainty established, though with the referent still vague, is that the young American princess "has it all." As James later makes clear, however, to Milly's mind there is still a deficiency in her life, for she has not yet experienced love.

When the two women journey to London to visit with an old school friend of Susan's, Milly enters a world for which she is wholly unfit. Though she becomes the object of attention and admiration within the English upper-class circle to which her hostess introduces her, she also becomes the target of an elaborate and base plan. Included in the circle of friends is a young couple who are in love but financially unable to marry, and who therefore keep their affection secret. The young woman in this pair, Kate Croy, becomes Milly's intimate friend; after learning two things—one, that Milly became acquainted with Merton Densher, the man Kate wishes to marry, during his stay in America, and two, that Milly is gravely ill—she sets in motion a plan. The design of Kate's plan is that Densher shall pretend to be in love with Milly, shall in fact marry her and become her heir, which will open the way to their future. The plan proceeds toward seeming success until another intimate of the circle, Lord Mark, proposes marriage to Milly. Since she can afford the luxury of refusing an English nobleman in the hope of marrying for love, Milly declines. Rebuffed, and suspicious that Milly intends to marry Densher, Lord Mark reveals to her his knowledge of the long-standing relationship Densher has maintained with Kate. At this Milly "turns her face to the wall," as Mrs. Stringham later describes her friend's passive response, and a short time after dies. In a grand gesture that affirms not only her noble qualities but also the increasing aura of sanctity engendered by her illness, Milly leaves her fortune to Densher. Shamed by the gesture, Densher refuses to allow himself and Kate to profit from Milly's death; he will marry Kate without the money or not at all. When he tells Kate they shall marry, but "[a]s we were," she turns toward the door with the final word: "We shall never be again as we were!"

Readers familiar with the novel will no doubt rebel at this truncated plot summary, which conveys nothing of the finely wrought and tenuous narrative lines on which James has constructed his story. In truth, no redaction of a James plot can ever do justice to the work since the author's style is singularly his; further, I have made no attempt to suggest the extent to which a number of the characters, beyond Kate and her lover, conspire for various reasons of their own in the deception of Milly Theale. The plot is here reduced to its essentials in order to focus attention on the interplay James develops between Milly's money and her illness, and on the sense of guilt that overshadows the ending and destroys all possibility of a future together for Kate and her lover.

Discussions of *The Wings of the Dove* almost always note that this is the only work in American literature that does not avoid the subject of tuberculosis and even dares to present a heroine who dies of the disease. James's position as an expatriate may have made this departure more imaginable for him, but it is also true that nowhere in the book is it stated explicitly that Milly Theale has TB. At one point Kate Croy even denigrates the idea, when Merton Densher raises the question by commenting, "Isn't consumption, taken in time, now curable?" (*Wings*, 214). Of course, by that point in the story we are not to be put off by Kate Croy, who has proven herself capable of almost any deceit, but Densher's question remains unanswered.

In truth, Milly's condition is referred to only by its symptoms and by subtle hints, such as her American doctor's instructions to seek a change of scene. The London doctor she consults, Sir Luke Strett, never offers any diagnosis, nor does he prescribe any treatment beyond advising her to escape the London winter, to worry about nothing, and "to live." When Mrs.

Stringham and her London friend, Mrs. Lowder, discuss Milly's illness and Sir Luke's reaction to it, Mrs. Stringham quotes him as saying "it *isn't* a case," which he later explains is not "*the* case" Milly had supposed, though his examination reveals "something else" (*Wings*, 245, 6). The "something else" is never clearly identified, but it would seem that Kate is attempting to minimize the unpleasantness associated with tuberculosis when she assures Densher that "[s]he won't die, she won't live, by inches. She won't smell, as it were, of drugs. She won't taste, as it were, of medicine. No one will know" (*Wings*, 215).

For critics, the question of what illness is being referred to is settled by James's frank admission, in *Notes of a Son and Brother* (1914), of the enormous effect on him of the death in 1870 of his young cousin, Minny Temple, from consumption. In 1892 his sister Alice died of breast cancer, which, from the descriptions of her death, had no doubt spread to her lung. It is possible that James had this in mind, that it is cancer that Milly Theale fears when she consults the London doctor and that, on examination, he finds is not "*the* case" but rather "something else"—consumption far enough advanced that there is nothing he can do but advise his young patient "to live," meaning, though he will not say it, to enjoy what life remains to her. For Milly there is but one thing for which she must still live, to know love.

Perhaps it was because Milly was the fictional representation of James's cousin Minny that he could not bring himself to name the disease, that he could only hint at it. As he points out in his preface, it was not the first time he had introduced into his novels a character who is terminally ill. Ralph Touchett in *The Portrait of a Lady* dies of a chronic lung illness, but Ralph is a secondary character in that novel. Still, the similarity between Ralph and Milly extends beyond their illness, for both are wealthy Americans involved with European schemers, and both arrive, in the course of their illness, at an understanding of the proper uses of wealth. Ralph leaves his money to the heroine of the novel, who is his cousin, and thereby enables her to fulfill her aspirations to independence. Milly leaves her money to Merton Densher, making possible for him a life of his own, with or without Kate Croy.

Milly Theale differs from Ralph Touchett, however, in that she shares more of Minny Temple's character, as James described it in a letter he wrote to his brother William only a short time after their cousin's death. There James admits that his grief at Minny's death is tempered by the awareness that "[h]er character may be almost literally said to have been without practical application to life." Minny was, he says, "the helpless victim and toy of her own intelligence. . . . She was restless . . . she was helpless . . . she was unpractical. . . . But what strikes me above all is how great and rare a benefit her life has been to those with whom she was associated."[21] Milly Theale, American "princess" and heiress, possesses all of Minny Temple's qualities as James describes them here, including the benefit to others gained from her life. That James considered himself to be the chief beneficiary of Minny's life, and death, is, at its base, the economic point on which his fictional equation of disease and wealth turns.

The family of Henry James was extremely gifted intellectually, but there existed among its members a peculiarly emotional bond of mind and body that was strengthened by a belief in a shared fund of health comparable to the inherited wealth that sustained them all. Just as Henry's extended tour of Europe as a youth affected his brother William's plans by drawing off a larger share of the family funds, so too Henry's good health at any given time was seen as a withdrawal on the family's joint deposit of health. The idea derived from the nineteenth-century belief in "neurasthenia," or nervous exhaustion, propounded by such figures in the new science of neurology as George M. Beard. According to this theory, nervous exhaustion occurred from making too great a drain on the finite amount of energy deposited in the human nervous system. It is possible to see in this peculiar notion (which is not all that peculiar given the care monied peoples of the time took with investments and all things economic) something of Emerson's theory of compensation, though somewhat skewed. Emerson had struggled through personal disasters of illness and death toward a belief that life is made up of polarities balanced by a law of nature that brings to each individual life equal amounts of good and evil. He made one of his first articulations of this belief in early manhood after his near blindness was corrected; undoubtedly the experience had taught him something of the compensatory nature of human sensory perception: "The whole of what we know is a system of compensation. . . . Every defect in one manner is made up in another. Every suffering is rewarded; every sacrifice is made up; every debt is paid" (Rusk, 115). In his literary theory Emerson also revealed a belief in compensation, extended to the plane of energy and power and broadened beyond individual resource, as when he describes, in "The Poet" (1844), "a great public power" from which the intellectual man draws energy beyond "his privacy of power as an individual man" (Whicher, 233).

The family of Henry James simply enlarged the Emersonian idea: its members drew on a shared, and finite, fund of health; the illness of any one member of the family was looked upon as a sort of deposit in the family bank from which the other members were drawing the benefit.[22] With this in mind, we can return to the letter James wrote to his brother at the time of his cousin's death and understand him when he speaks of "the gradual change and reversal of our relations: I slowly crawling from weakness and inaction and suffering [James had experienced an attack of typhus while traveling abroad] into strength and hope: she sinking out of brightness and youth into decline and death" (*Letters*, 224). Like Ralph Touchett, the TB sufferer in *The Portrait of a Lady* who gives up his inheritance to make possible his cousin's chance at life, Minny Temple, to James's mind, had sacrificed her health for his.

This idea about Minny's illness and death burned in James's consciousness for years; as he says in the preface to *Wings*, "I can scarce remember
the time when the situation on which this long-drawn fiction mainly rests
was not vividly present to me" (v). Having long projected "a certain sort of
young American as more the 'heir of all the ages' than any other young person
whatever," he writes, ". . . here was a chance to confer on some such figure
a supremely touching value" (ix). His use of the word *value*, which has
decidedly economic connotations, cannot be ignored despite whatever other
meaning it is meant to convey when applied to the young American. For one
thing, it is exactly the word Milly uses when the full realization of her position
comes to her: "[W]ouldn't her value, for the man who should marry her, be
precisely in the ravage of her disease? *She* mightn't last, but her money
would" (*Wings*, 267). Although such calculation could never be attached to
the Emerson marriage, James, whose father was acquainted with Ralph
Waldo Emerson, knew full well that Emerson's writing career had been
made possible by the small fortune he inherited at his first wife's death from
tuberculosis. The opportunity James now has to confer "value" on the image
of Minny, whose death, like that of Ellen Emerson, seemed to him to have
made possible his own career, coincides with his decision to free himself from
the tyranny of literary magazines. It is as if his freedom to do so were another
part of his inheritance from Minny, part of the family store of health-wealth
on which he continues to draw.

As might be expected, especially from so highly principled a mind as that
of Henry James, he felt a sense of guilt at having benefited from Minny's
deposit of her illness in the family fund. The guilt comes through in the
preface, where James cannot resist the suggestion that his heroine contributes to her own betrayal. Though in Milly Theale James had created a perfect
dove of innocence, he seems, in the preface, to dwell on her culpability in the
plot by which she is undone. Once having decided on Milly for the dovelike
role, he tells us that his business was to watch, "as the fond parent watches
a child perched, for its first riding-lesson, in the saddle," but knowing that "a
creature with her security hanging so by a hair, couldn't but fall somehow
into some abysmal trap" (*Wings*, ix). This image, of course, echoes James's
letter to William in which he speaks of the inevitability, had she lived, of
Minny's downfall. But in the preface the inevitability of Milly's fall does not
entirely absolve her, in James's mind, of all guilt. He refers to her as one of the
Rhine maidens and may have had in mind Richard Wagner's *Das Rheingold*
(1854), in which the Rhine maidens who guard the golden ring set in motion
a great economic disaster by their sexual provocations. Milly's existence
would create yet another kind of havoc, James decides, "very much that
whirlpool movement of the waters produced by the sinking of a big vessel or
the failure of a great business" (*Wings*, x). Despite these "communities of
doom," he claims to have seen the disaster "much more prepared *for* my
vessel of sensibility than by her—the work of other hands (though with her

own imbrued too, after all, in the measure of their never not being, in some direction, generous and extravagant, and thereby provoking)" (*Wings*, x). Try as he may, James cannot seem to eschew the economic imagery. Nor can he view Milly as entirely innocent; he must point to her culpability, even if parenthetically.

In retrospect, James sees his heroine provoking, even tempting others, by her great wealth and her desire to have it "all," into "promoting her illusion" that her love for Merton Densher is returned. Of these others James is also keenly aware (no doubt having felt some kinship to them); he justifies having delayed his heroine's appearance until—using two books of the first volume to accomplish it—he had set the stage for the intrigue to come: "If one had seen that her stricken state was but half her case, the correlative half being the state of others as affected by her . . . then I was free to choose, as it were, the half with which I should begin" (*Wings*, x).

"[T]hen I was free to choose" is the operative phrase by which we are made aware that a great deal about this book speaks of James's own sense of having been drawn into Milly's orbit. Only for him it is more truly Minny Temple's orbit, the circumference of which was formed, as James says of her image so long held in memory, "to make the wary adventurer walk round and round it" (*Wings*, v). That image, rooted in the memory of his cousin's death, gave rise to a subject matter, illness, that, he claims, had "a charm that invited and mystified . . . it might have a great deal to give, but would probably ask for equal services in return, and would collect this debt to the last shilling" (*Wings*, v). It is not possible to miss the connection in James's mind between this mysterious and tempting subject matter, ill health, and money. It would appear that his use of tuberculosis as a metaphor for the economic freedom that Milly becomes acutely conscious of only when it is threatened, is in some way related to his own expanded artistic economy, a kind of full-blown literary consciousness the luxury of which may have been strongly reminiscent of the impracticality of the real Milly, Minny Temple.

Having scorned the profession of a Susan Stringham and turned his back on the well-paying periodicals, James claims to have known a freedom in writing *The Wings of the Dove* that allowed him to choose at every point what he most wished to do. As the text bears witness, what he most wished was to compose in a manner that might be termed spendthrift in its discursiveness. Indeed, in his letters to William Dean Howells at the time James refers repeatedly to the subject of word limitations and speaks of his fears that *Wings* is too long. Against those who might complain at this and at the novel's resulting length, James defends himself by admitting that he expects "attention of perusal" from his readers, adding: "The enjoyment of a work of art, the acceptance of an irresistible illusion, constituting, to my sense, our highest experience of 'luxury,' is not greatest, by my consequent measure, when the work asks for as little attention as possible" (*Wings*, xxi). Clearly the connection between health and wealth established within the novel extends to the benefit of artistic freedom James feels he has gained by at last committing to art the tribute to his cousin he had long wished to make, even though it required that he "look so straight in the face and so closely to cross-question that idea of making one's protagonist 'sick' " (*Wings*, vi). Whatever it was about Minny that fascinated him while at the same time making him wholly uneasy about her ability to get through life without encountering, even provoking, the kind of disaster he invents for Milly Theale, had to do with Minny's character being "without practical application to life." The risk he took in exercising his creative freedom with such a character was that the subject might, at the last, be equally without practical application to art.

This text has received wide critical attention, and I have made no attempt here to add to it a detailed *explication*; my intent is to concentrate on James's use of tuberculosis in the working out of plot. In that regard the conjunction of great wealth with the disease seems not only to follow other economically based references in James's works but to equate the power of wealth with another kind of power, the often manipulative power of the ill to shape the lives of others in lieu of their own. It is interesting to note that, though most critics have not taken Milly Theale to task as James does in his preface, one who has finds her "doomed as much by her own psychology [which makes her unable to cope with life] as by her illness."[23] This criticism, as we shall see, echoes Emerson's of Thoreau and underscores the risk involved in introducing a protagonist who is sick from the moment of presentation and for whom justification must be offered. Emerson's eulogistic portrayal of his friend's life reflected his disappointment at Thoreau's renunciation of ambition and desire; James's eulogistic portrayal of his tubercular cousin is that of someone unable to fashion her own life but who ultimately shapes the lives of others by dying.

Milly Theale gradually fades from the book that is ostensibly her story; as her illness progresses, the antiheroine Kate Croy comes more and more to the fore. Indeed, as Kate has promised, Milly does not betray signs of her illness by sight or smell; she retreats into her rented villa in Venice until the day when she "turns her face to the wall" and, understanding at last the full extent of the betrayal she has suffered, ceases to follow Sir Luke's advice "to live." In scrutinizing his own text at the time of preparing the New York Edition, James notes the "indirection" with which he treats the subject of Milly's illness. His style "resorts for relief," he admits, "whenever it can, to some kinder, some merciful indirection: all as if to approach her circuitously, deal with her at second hand, as an unspotted princess is ever dealt with; the pressure all round her kept easy for her, the sounds, the movements regulated, the forms and ambiguities made charming" (*Wings*, xxii). The charm with which James masks the forms and ambiguities of illness (the ambiguity revealing itself even by the need to clear his princess of clinical associations to tuberculosis by claiming she is "unspotted") arises from the employment of his art in such a way as to give free rein to the indirection of metaphor, and thus to assert his own economic and artistic freedom.

= TB and the Power of the Individual =

Though I have identified the idea of a contagion of indolence specifically with a twentieth-century literary work, O'Neill's *Long Day's Journey into Night*, it is so intrinsically a part of the American psyche to expect everyone to demonstrate a high degree of motivation that the concept can hardly be considered a contemporary phenomenon. One reason for the silence of American writers on the subject of tuberculosis is undoubtedly connected to a sense of individual failure felt by its victims. Hidden behind the mythology that developed around the disease in the nineteenth century seems to have been the fear of inadequacy and even of moral bankruptcy suggested by becoming afflicted with a disease from which one usually could not recover. In *The Great Gatsby* (1925) F. Scott Fitzgerald's narrator, Nick Carraway, realizes "that there was no difference between men, in intelligence or race, so profound as the difference between the sick and the well."[24] This difference must have been especially apparent in nineteenth-century America, where the perception of what constituted a self-reliant individual involved health and strength, a perception that would have contributed to the imaging of the tubercular patient as a female, a child, or a sensitive, artistic male. The drive to succeed in an economic and political environment that presented little hindrance to the exercise of individual power pushed many to the limits of their physical strength while impoverishing them spiritually, a condition of which nineteenth-century New England's latter-day Puritans were especially aware. The American emphasis on success and on the need to achieve it to prove one's self-sufficiency in a capitalist society would also have contributed to making the tubercular patient feel deficient, for one could not succeed in a competitive society if one's strength and time were limited. Neither could such an individual invest heavily in the effort to regain health—thus fulfilling the responsibility of cooperating in one's recovery—if the effort seemed doomed by heredity. The played-out New England farmlands inherited by fourth- or fifth-generation Americans, the failure of the national economy in 1837, and Thoreau's sense that he would not live to achieve the only kind of success he valued, as a writer, all combined in the making of *Walden*. An apologia offered by an individual destined to that peculiar democracy of the sick, *Walden* takes a belligerent stance against an economic system that later made possible the corporate world of Standard Oil. Whether there is in this a veiled fear of his own inadequacy in such a social order, a fear wrought by the knowledge of his "inherited" disease, is hard to say, but in his final days

Thoreau's letters reveal that he was much in need of reassurance that his writing had not been "in vain" (Harding, 457, 460).

Emerson's eulogy for Thoreau contains one obvious outburst of disappointment at his friend's chosen path: "I so much regret the loss of his rare powers of action, that I cannot help counting it a fault in him that he had no ambition. Wanting this, instead of engineering for all America, he was the captain of a huckleberry-party. Pounding beans is good to the end of pounding empires one of these days; but if, at the end of years, it is still only beans!" (Whicher, 393). By sheer good fortune Emerson had recovered from his attack of tuberculosis, and there may be in this outburst a hint of smugness and superiority at having had sufficient spiritual power to overcome his illness. From this perspective Thoreau's failure to regain his health could be viewed as a refusal to cooperate in his own recovery, to fulfill his role as a sick but recovering member of the family. Such a view might even have led Emerson to see this refusal as yet another instance of that irritating intractability in his friend that he also deplored. In 1843 he confided his annoyance and disappointment, and perhaps his fear, to his journal: "Young men like H.T. owe us a new world & they have not acquitted the debt," Emerson wrote, adding prophetically, "for the most part, such die young, & so dodge the fulfillment."[25] Of the two men, Emerson was more in tune with the progressive economic mood of the country. His attitude must have made it all the more difficult for him to accept Thoreau's reluctance to engineer "for all America" when, in 1846, while Thoreau was still lingering at Walden's shores, Harvard College proposed a school of practical science, one aim of which was to provide the nation with skilled engineers (Brown, 24). The reality was that, like his health, the provincial New England that Thoreau hoped to see return was beyond recovery, and he was never at ease in the commercial and industrial society that had replaced it.

The hierarchy of spiritual over material values established by the New England transcendentalists in the years when tuberculosis was rampant in that region was an attempt to wed metaphysics to free enterprise, all in the interest of bolstering the status of the self-reliant individual capable of subjecting the natural universe to his or her gaze and extracting from it knowledge and power. This ideational power of the individual Emerson set over against the communal power of the social reformers, those who would seek to gain knowledge of nature, and especially human nature, through the observations of the scientific and the societal eye. To the builders of cooperative communes—and they were many in nineteenth-century America— crime, disease, and poverty were all social ills traceable to the competitive spirit that fed the economy, but to Emerson and Thoreau they were the result of a misplaced emphasis on the products of that economy, on the "things" that "ride mankind."

Tuberculosis, which they could lay to no known cause, offered nineteenth-century American writers an apt image of spirit triumphing over matter, an image Henry James seriously questioned. Writing after Koch's discovery, James had the benefit of a greater medical understanding of the disease, but he also had the benefit of having seen at first hand what could happen to America's peculiar brand of spirituality when brought into play on the international scene. The spiritual refinement that earlier was believed to accompany the advance of tuberculosis is demonstrated to the fullest in Milly Theale's final abdication of her wealth along with her fondest desire. But she has paid a high price for her spirituality, and one can seriously question, as James ultimately did, both her motives and her culpability in the events that overtake her. As always in James, the exercise of individual power, which he viewed as a perverted use of economic freedom (and which Emerson tried to disguise as the evidence of increased spirit), is fraught with peril. Of all James's ill-fated heroines, Milly Theale is the most tragic if for no other reason than that she is the most representative of the thousands like her in nineteenth-century America, male and female, who, by virtue of being Americans, were each potential heirs and heiresses of the ages but whose freedom and economic power were thwarted by tuberculosis. Though cholera swept the nation three times in that same century, tuberculosis was by far the greater destroyer of American hope by its indiscriminate attack on all social and economic levels. Indeed, the scourge of tuberculosis wrought a kind of equality in America undreamed of in a capitalistic philosophy.

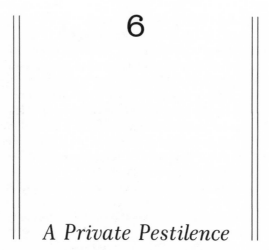

6

A Private Pestilence

ON 9 DECEMBER 1979 THE WORLD HEALTH ORGANIZATION
officially declared the global eradication of smallpox. One year later the first
cases of acquired immune deficiency syndrome (AIDS) were diagnosed in
the Western world. Seen in relation to each other these two events indicate
one thing clearly—that epidemic diseases are with us now as they were in
the Middle Ages, in the time of the European Renaissance, and in the Age
of Enlightenment. And given the close proximity of the two events, it would
seem that in human history the vacancy left by the conquering of one epidemical "scourge" (in the value-laden language of the Middle Ages) will be almost
immediately filled by another. To succumb to this seeming inevitability with
resignation and a sense of doom, however, would be to renounce one of the
great lessons of modern medicine—that epidemics are part of human history, are not of supernatural origin, and are therefore susceptible to human
correction.

As some of our romance writers have tried to warn us, the problem
created by this modern, rationalistic mode of thinking is the reliance it fosters

125

on medical science and the impatience it breeds when—as in the case of the AIDS virus—a "cure" is not quickly forthcoming. For a time, while the general population is not threatened, this impatience may be held in check; but with the passage of time and a widening of the epidemical horizon, a greater sense of urgency stimulates the desire to identify and segregate those who present the most likely threat. We have seen in earlier chapters how this urgency, justifiable in medical terms, can be carried over into the social realm and individual rights set aside in the interests of a societal end. Many have feared such a reaction in countries where AIDS is especially virulent, but thus far there has been only one such extreme response to the AIDS crisis, in Cuba. In this communist nation, whose island status affords easy immigration control, the government has instituted a mandatory program of testing for all citizens as well as for those who seek entry into the country. Treatment for those citizens who test positive follows the model of the earlier leprosariums in its long-term isolation of patients, even those who are still symptom-free. Probably the most repressive AIDS program undertaken by any nation, the principle behind the Cuban approach is that the AIDS patient must sacrifice individual rights in the interests of the entire society.[1]

At the other end of the political spectrum, there exists in the United States, where immigration is a historical fact of national life and individual freedom a political given, a potential for surveillance and repression greater than ever before in the nation's history, given the extensive bureaucratic use of computerized information. To date, such surveillance has remained minimal, but as medical answers to AIDS continue to elude researchers the possibility of its implementation becomes more real. At present the United States is in a transitional phase, moving away from its earlier willful ignorance about AIDS toward a more vigilant posture; inevitably, the nation is simultaneously attempting to adjust the scales in which it balances individual rights and societal needs.

= "Living with AIDS" =

In 1989 *Daedalus*, a journal of scholarly opinion that enjoys high international repute, devoted a double issue to the subject of AIDS under the title "Living with AIDS." Its aim was to dispel the idea that the world is simply marking time until a cure is developed for this disease. Eliminating AIDS, the journal pointed out, "would require the mandatory testing of the six billion and more people in the world coupled with immediate, mandatory treatment of all who were HIV positive. Even if the astronomical costs of such an effort could be borne, the logistics of achieving mandatory worldwide testing and treatment seem insuperably difficult."[2] In lieu of such infeasible measures, *Daedalus* posited education about the disease as the world's best hope for curbing its spread while science continues its search for cause and cure. Educative

approaches were slow to start in the United States, largely owing to a governmental policy of neglect and a general belief in the ability of medicine to
dispel the danger. As hope for success in conquering the virus scientifically
has dimmed, however, the United States has dropped its early "see no evil"
blindness toward the AIDS threat and adopted more aggressive and, at times,
exclusionary methods to contain it. To date almost every such step has been
viewed as a misstep by some segment of the population; perhaps the most
damning argument comes from Randy Shilts, author of *And the Band Played
On* (1987), who contends that the health beauracracy in the United States
failed its mission and allowed the epidemic to spread.[3] Before examining that
argument and the response it has brought from one segment of the AIDS-
affected community, a brief description of the disease (still in many ways a
mystery) is in order.

= Acquired Immune Deficiency =
Syndrome

Acquired immune deficiency syndrome is caused by an infectious microor-
ganism, a virus called the human immunodeficiency virus type 1 (HIV-1).[4]
Its place of origin remains unclear, but cases of an unknown viral disease
were first noted in Africa in the 1970s and in the United States in 1980.
These two nations remain the epicenters for the disease, though AIDS special-
ists predict that Asia will soon rival them in incidence. Infection brings on a
slow, progressive degenerative disease of both the immune and the central
nervous systems. Because HIV is a retrovirus—the class of viruses that implant themselves in cells and cause disease much later—seven to ten years
usually intervene between infection and the onset of symptoms, during which
time the virus may be transmitted. Currently it is believed that the AIDS
virus has been infecting people (and possibly animals) for a very long time,
but that it has only become an observable phenomenon in our time. (The
oldest documented case of AIDS is that of a British sailor whose death in
1959 was a medical mystery until tests performed in 1985 on tissue samples
saved from his body proved he suffered from AIDS.)[5]

HIV infection occurs from the transfer of bodily fluids: blood, semen,
saliva, tears, urine, spinal fluid, breast milk, and vaginal secretions. Its primary routes of transmission are sexual contact with an infected person,
exposure to infected blood or blood products, and passage from an infected
mother to her infant before or during birth. The population groups most
at risk include homosexuals and bisexuals (though in Africa the virus is
transmitted heterosexually, as is increasingly the case in the United States),
intravenous drug users, those in need of blood transfusions, offspring of
infected mothers, and those involved in the care of AIDS patients. The disease
is always fatal.

AIDS destroys the body's immune system by obliterating the T-cells that are vital to the protection of the body against other infections, both viral and bacterial. At present only one drug is licensed by the U.S. Food and Drug Administration (FDA) for treatment of HIV infection, the drug known as AZT (azidothymidine), which postpones the development of full-blown AIDS in HIV-infected persons. There is no cure, and no vaccine. Factors militating against the development of a vaccine include the following: there are many different HIV strains, which exhibit various mutations in each infected person's body; previous vaccines were facilitated by our ability to study the nature of the immune response in individuals who had recovered without treatment, but there are no fully recovered AIDS patients; there are no animal models on which to draw.

That AIDS causes so many varied medical problems also complicates its treatment. A patient with HIV infection may exhibit, among numerous other ailments, pneumocystis carinii pneumonia, the most common opportunistic infection among patients in industrialized countries; toxoplasmosis; gastrointestinal infections; cytomegalovirus, which can cause blindness; herpesvirus, a skin disease; candida, or thrush mouth, fungus; and Kaposi's sarcoma, a type of cancer characterized by purple skin lesions. (The longer a treated AIDS patient remains alive, the more prone he or she is to developing cancer at other sites.) As the patient population widens to include more women and intravenous drug users, this list of symptoms is lengthening because in each group the disease manifests itself differently. The problem created by a rigid definition of AIDS based on the first group to develop the disease, gay males, is the failure of some doctors to recognize certain other conditions as being AIDS-related.

Despite the overwhelming ignorance about the disease at the time of its discovery, the worldwide medical community has been remarkably diligent in its research efforts; more has been learned about the virus in a scant eight to ten years than about any other microbe, including those that have been known to science for a century. New knowledge is added almost daily, encouraging the belief that the disease will someday be fully known and that the discovery of its cause and the development of treatments and a cure are not far off. Nevertheless, the World Health Organization has predicted the staggering figure, 40 million, as the number of people in the world who will be infected by the year 2000. As that year approaches and the figures continue to mount toward the devastating forecast, the principal mysteries still facing researchers are these: (1) Why does AIDS spread faster in some countries than in others? (2) Why do some people live for years after infection while others die quickly? (3) Where does the virus enter the body, and how does infection begin? (4) Why is the body's immune response ineffective against HIV?[6]

Because it is not a single disease but a syndrome, and precisely because so much about its spread remains mysterious, AIDS has encouraged surveillance both of the disease and of its victims, a surveillance characterized by vigilance and detachment. The belief that the disease only affects a marginal segment of the population (that is, homosexuals and intravenous drug users) encourages a desire to be vigilant, to keep an eye on "them" to see that "they" do not spread it to "us." But a concomitant detachment, the belief that those who are not part of that marginal population will remain unaffected, has allowed the disease to spread. To a degree, this detachment has also encouraged a reluctance to take aggressive measures against the disease because more can be learned about it by observing its progress. That kind of detachment has resulted in the introduction of the disease into nonmarginal segments of the general population. For example, a laissez-faire attitude toward those in the health fields has resulted in transmission of the virus from an infected dentist to a number of his patients, and the Centers for Disease Control (CDC) is now attempting to write new guidelines to protect patients from health-care workers infected with the AIDS virus. As if in support of this intent, a survey funded by the Department of Health and Human Services showed a majority of doctors and nurses favor mandatory testing of health-care workers. The same survey also revealed that a majority favor mandatory AIDS testing for all surgical patients and pregnant women, provided results of the tests were used only for the purpose of advising treatment. These opinions were interpreted as a shift within the medical community away from a focus on individual rights, based on a perceived need to approach AIDS from the same standard of public health that is applied to other communicable diseases.[7] But at a meeting of the American Medical Association (AMA) held after the survey results were released, AMA members voted overwhelmingly in opposition to testing of health-care workers and patients, and the American Nurses Association voted the same way. It remains to be seen if this stand by the medical profession will be reflected in governmental policies and procedures, or if conflict will develop between medicine and government.

AIDS is a test of American society and its political and moral beliefs unlike any that has occurred in this century. Social upheaval in the 1960s and 1970s placed great stress on societal bonds, but Americans drew deeply on common goals and transcended that danger. AIDS, however, offers no common goal other than its cure—which remains elusive—and the realization of the best hope that medicine can offer, the ability to live with it. These goals are difficult to accept and integrate into thought patterns conditioned to instant remedy. Another great difficulty is the need to reconceive the idea of public health. Up to this point the "public" has referred to the citizens of "mainstream" America whose health needs are being served by government agencies. Faced with the spreading AIDS epidemic, however, the more politically active segment of the population most threatened, the gay community, has urged a redefinition of the term "public" to include those groups and individuals considered marginal. In large part, the growing awareness of this need for redefinition comes from the realization that this disease will not be "conquered" by vigilant surveillance of the marginal "others" in society, and that detachment must give way to an expanded collective perception that includes these "others" within the national social parameters.

A full exploration of AIDS-related political decisions and policies is beyond the scope of this study; but they include certain attitudes and philosophical positions that inform our intellectual and cultural life and are reflected in our literature. To begin with, in America AIDS presents special problems of restriction in that it takes us into the areas of privacy that have been protected by law from public scrutiny and legal control. The use of some drugs is illegal, but we do not (usually) invade peoples' homes to see if they are using them; neither do we invade their bedrooms to see if they are engaging in unsafe sex. Public health officials therefore have a very difficult time trying to protect the physical well-being of the nation without inhibiting individual freedom. In this epidemic the fate of the community depends upon the private behavior of its individual members; the question then becomes one of either surveillance or education aimed at altering private behavior where it threatens public health.

This is not to say that legal measures are not or have not been brought into play, but the pattern thus far established is one in which stern measures that provoke strong opposition are modified. Precedent exists for some of the measures taken; for instance, laws prohibiting spitting on public thoroughfares were passed under the impetus of the antituberculosis sanitary movement. The intersecting of private and public interests is especially apparent in the area of health and accident insurance. Laws mandating the use of seat belts in automobiles, requiring motorcycle riders to wear helmets, banning smoking in most public places, and prohibiting from driving those who have partaken of more than a certain amount of alcoholic beverages, all have their origins in the need to curb the prohibitive insurance costs incurred by victims of these actions. Insurance companies are already trying to avoid the high costs involved in AIDS care. Since legal prohibition of certain behaviors, principally sexual behavior, is impossible, individuals who come under what are termed high-risk categories by reason of occupation or other affiliations thought to reflect unorthodox sexual practices often are denied medical insurance or are faced with extremely high premium costs. Determinations of who is considered high-risk may now be made legally in some states through AIDS tests administered to applicants for medical insurance; while this will deter some companies from using less objective methods of screening applicants, it will likely deny insurance to those found to be carrying the virus.

Some medico-legal actions taken in response to the AIDS crisis, such as the closing of public bathhouses, a measure also taken under earlier epidemic conditions, and the screening of blood donors, have not met with serious resistance. The screening of blood donors did arouse the ire of one ethnic group, the Haitians, who were singled out (as they were in the 1790s when yellow fever was believed by many to have been imported by immigrants fleeing that island's revolution) and excluded from blood donation because of the high rate of HIV infection on that island. Reacting to their protests, the federal government lifted the ban and intensified its testing efforts instead. Similarly, after two years of debate AIDS was removed from the list of illnesses that prevented individuals from entering the United States. (Other diseases whose sufferers are denied entry are syphilis, gonorrhea, leprosy, and tuberculosis.) This action, undertaken on the advice of the Public Health Service, was later challenged by the Justice Department, which cited, among other reasons for its disagreement, the receipt of thousands of letters protesting the change. At present the position of the Justice Department prevails, and AIDS has been returned to the list. Clearly, the government is making and revising policy not always on the basis of medical evidence but often in reaction to the loudest voices raised.

Organizations representing the gay community have opposed proposals by the CDC for broad confidential testing on a voluntary basis because they see a potential for persecution in any such plan. These same organizations were especially fearful of attempts by conservative politicians during the Reagan administration to use testing as a means of identifying and restricting the movements of individuals who were HIV-positive. Prison officials attempting to deal with the escalation in the number of AIDS-infected inmates have run afoul of the American Civil Liberties Union, which has successfully prevented mandatory testing of prisoners and isolation of those known to be infected. Even the dead, though they have no civil rights, figure in the national dilemma of AIDS and the need to acquire knowledge about it. New York City now routinely includes a test for the disease in all autopsies performed by its chief medical examiner's office; the results are used for statistical research and to inform survivors of potential contact danger. Nationally, organ or tissue donations now must await testing for the virus as a result of a case in which four recipients of body parts from one infected donor contracted the disease. The nation is involved in an educative process by which it learns, almost daily, something new about the progress of this epidemic, as well as about the ways in which attempts to curb it often conflict with those liberties guaranteed by a free society.

An awareness of this conflict is reflected in the general consensus, among those who write on the topic, that public health officials may only rightfully hope to pursue educative means to protect the general health of the nation from AIDS. A complicating factor, however, is the belief of some that any educative approach on this subject must include the teaching of moral values. Although this position is held for the most part by religious groups, there are also those in the medical field who see a need to support calls for greater morality because of the danger posed by the disease.[8] The other side of this coin is that those social educators who oppose the translation of medical issues into moral or religious ones often fail to carry their concern beyond the obvious (such as offering support for the distribution of condoms or clean intravenous needles) and ignore the private pain felt by the infected, who are, and continue to be, morally stigmatized and ostracized. Clearly, not even the educative approach to combating this disease is without dilemma.

The issue of private rights versus public good is not, of course, the main reason for the government's slowness—or failure, in Randy Shilts's eyes—to recognize the danger of AIDS. Shilts believes this inertia had more to do with the coincidence of the disease appearing during the high-flying years of Reagan prosperity, when public officials were motivated to ignore anything that might stem the swelling economic tide or place too great a demand on government funds (324). But there may also have been a reluctance within the medical bureaucracy to repeat some of the errors of the recent and not so recent past. For in modern American history the track record of the Public Health Service in handling epidemical situations is not a good one. If anything, there had been an overreaction by the government to two threats to public health in the recent past, neither of which could be compared for gravity with the threat posed by AIDS.

= Public Health Emergencies =

Interestingly, both of these threats to public health occurred in 1976, the year of the bicentennial of the United States of America. Some epidemiologists also connect the beginning of the AIDS epidemic in this country to the same year, seeing the arrival in New York Harbor of ships and crews from 55 nations as a causative event (Shilts, 3). Whatever the significance of these coeval events, which history may yet reveal, reliable medical sources predicted an outbreak of swine flu in 1976 similar in magnitude to the epidemic of 1918, which had resulted in the deaths of more than 600,000 Americans. As the CDC prepared the formulation of that year's influenza vaccine, it took careful note of these predictions and rushed to produce a vaccine that would protect the greatest number of citizens, especially those in the high-risk categories, the very young, the aged, and the chronically ill. Pressured by the fear of seeing history repeat itself in another influenza epidemic, the government allowed vaccine manufacturers only a short time to develop the vaccine. The manufacturers, prevented from doing adequate testing and fearing that the vaccine might itself cause illness or death for which they would have to accept responsibility, lobbied Congress, which enacted special legislation indemnifying manufacturers for possible legal awards above a certain amount. The government moved forward rapidly, and a vaccine was produced and administered to millions. Perhaps it was inevitable, but there were serious side effects from the vaccine, including the occurrence in over 100 of those vaccinated of the paralytic disease Guillain-Barre syndrome. This unforeseen development brought the immunization program to an end, and the government had to cover the manufacturers' liability.

That same year at a state convention of the American Legion held in Philadelphia, a group of conventioneers became ill with a strange type of pneumonia. It later proved to be a known strain of the disease, but one that had never occurred in a large number of people all at one time; nonetheless, it was far from being an epidemic, despite the 29 deaths that resulted. The government, however, spurred on by the publicity afforded the outbreak and by the efforts of Sen. Richard Schweiker of Pennsylvania, established an emergency fund for health research that later became a source of political wrangling when the AIDS emergency did not qualify for access to it. Oddly, establishment of the fund did not include a definition of what constituted a health emergency that would warrant access to it, and therefore no one had a clear idea of when the money might be spent. If Legionnaires' disease, as the convention-connected pneumonia came to be known, with 29 deaths to its record could constitute an emergency calling for the establishment of public funds, what could be said of a threat the size of AIDS? Yet the government delayed, and even with the passage in 1983 of the Health Emergency Act, no provision was made for the needed care and coordination of services for AIDS patients.[9]

Although this record of mismanagement had the potential to affect the majority of Americans, one minority group had even greater cause to doubt the wisdom of the country's public health administration. Still within the memory of many African-Americans is the infamous syphilis experiment undertaken by the PHS in 1932: 412 black male sharecroppers in Tuskegee, Alabama, were made subjects of a study designed to observe the progress of syphilis through all stages of its ravaging of the human body. Denied knowledge of their illness—they were told that they had "bad blood"—the men were also denied treatment even after penicillin had proved effective against syphilis.[10] Terminated in 1972, the study, which became a matter of public record a short time later, has raised deeply troubling questions about the ethics involved in medical observation techniques, especially when directed toward members of minority or marginal groups. So damaging has knowledge of this study been to the confidence of African-Americans in governmental health agencies that some within that community, which has a high incidence of AIDS, believe that AIDS is a deliberate attempt by the government to eliminate them in this country.[11] In recognition of this lack of trust, the PHS sponsored a symposium in June 1991 to discuss the Tuskegee study with researchers, ethicists, doctors, and other health-care officials and to examine its effects on the relationship between the medical profession and African-Americans.

Unfortunately, the highly publicized record of sometime neglect and sometime overvigilance obscures the record of the efficient and well-managed health care more routinely provided by the PHS. But it has been enough to cause the PHS to experience some conflicted reactions as it has faced the spreading AIDS epidemic. Perhaps it wanted to avoid the kind of negative response Ibsen portrays in *An Enemy of the People* (1882) to physicians who issue warnings of impending civic disaster. Nevertheless, if PHS administrators had reviewed the agency's recent record in meeting medical emergencies they might have noted some similarities: the sudden appearance among the victims of Legionnaires' disease of a pneumonia never before seen in such proportions, and the pneumocystis carinii pneumonia that so often is the first symptom of AIDS; the movement of swine flu from animal to human populations, and the theory, one of many, that AIDS originally had appeared among the green monkey population in Africa; and the erroneous belief held by many that the sexually transmittable disease AIDS is like syphilis in that it is rampant within a minority of the citizenry because of their lack of morals. (In fact, though it can be sexually transmitted, AIDS is not a venereal disease but a disease of the blood.) Rather than risk another debacle by moving too quickly in any one direction, taking the long view and hoping for a cure may have seemed the better medical course. In retrospect, however, it appears that the prevailing response was rooted in a fear already familiar from the time of the yellow fever epidemics in the earliest days of our national history: the fear of government that officially admitting to the presence of epidemical disease would bring on economic and political disaster.

= AIDS and Previous Epidemics =

Governmental inaction is not the only similarity between the attitudes and beliefs arising from the AIDS epidemic and those associated with the other epidemics discussed in this book. New York's John Cardinal O'Connor may not see himself as a kind of twentieth-century pastor-physician, nor has he thus far shown himself to be in the forefront of medical thinking on AIDS (as Cotton Mather was on the subject of smallpox inoculation). But he has not hesitated to make known his understanding of the disease—for which more than one newspaper has followed in the tradition of eighteenth-century Boston's *New-England Courant* and aimed anticlerical barbs at the cardinal. In literary terms, the ambiguity in Hawthorne's "Lady Eleanore's Mantle" about the source of Boston's smallpox epidemic—whether it was foreign or domestic—is ultimately not so important as the connection the author draws between the epidemic and the spirit of revolution abroad in America at the time. Similarly, political and social revolution presaged the appearance of AIDS in America, stirring in the minds of many the often unconscious view of epidemical disease as divine punishment for human transgression of the boundaries of acceptable behavior. Further, Hawthorne's imaging of a woman as the carrier of a loathsome disease touches on his century's fear of the syphilitic prostitute in the same way that our century has fastened on the image of the AIDS victim as sexually or socially deviant. And as we have already seen, John Edgar Wideman makes the connection, in his story

"Fever," between epidemic disease and social unrest even in contemporary society.

Still more similarities exist. People on the fringes of society, the socially marginalized, are just as easily stigmatized today as were blacks in the yellow fever epidemics or, more recently, in the 1932 PHS syphilis experiment. Gays became identified with AIDS in the first years of its occurrence because of its initial detection in male homosexuals. In fact, so firm was the association in the minds of doctors that the disease was for a time called gay-related immune deficiency. Not until July 1982, at a Washington, D.C. meeting of representatives of various health and government agencies, the blood services industry, and gay community groups, was the name by which we now know the disease affixed.

The present nomenclature for the virus indicates a syndrome of acquired rather than congenitally or chemically induced problems of the immune system, and though the name implies that the disease is caused by a source outside the body, its exact etiology remains a mystery. The name change, however, did little to alter the attitude of most Americans. The statement by John Pintard at the time of the 1832 cholera epidemic in New York City, in which he expressed gratitude that the disease was confined to "the lower classes of intemperate dissolute and filthy people" and was sparing the city's "regular householders," reflects an attitude all too common in the current AIDS epidemic. Only recently, with the extension of the disease into the heterosexual community of what many consider to be "regular householders" (or members of the "general population," as the official language has it), has there been a gradual attempt to consider the epidemic as something that might be of concern to those who do not inhabit the margins of American society. Despite the widening of attention, and because the disease has been so closely associated with homosexuality and drug use in the minds of most Americans, the gay community has assumed a position of leadership and has taken upon itself the task, in ways that shall be discussed presently, of reshaping the general perception of the disease and those it afflicts.

Of the economic dimension to the AIDS epidemic much has been said and written, especially with regard to the need for greater funding, through both public and private agencies, to make possible more research, to provide health care, less costly drugs, and other services to those who have the disease, to facilitate program grants distributed by individual states, and so forth. An additional, though not so readily apparent, international aspect of the problem involves the notion of a kind of residual fund of health from which all nations draw. Careful perusal of the two issues of *Daedalus* devoted to AIDS makes one aware of the global dimensions, explored by many of the writers, that move AIDS beyond national considerations, indeed, beyond an epidemic to a pandemic level. One writer observes that AIDS provides a pragmatic foundation for the belief that nations are interdependent in the area of health because the health of humanity may be thought of as a common resource—a view that seems remarkably close to James's health-wealth economy underlying his approach to tuberculosis in *The Wings of the Dove*, and that establishes yet another link between this and other epidemics.[12]

= AIDS in the Public Eye =

A marked dissimilarity between the AIDS crisis and earlier epidemics in America is the assertive action taken by one affected group. Acting in response to what it perceives as a pattern of neglect on the part of government agencies, the medical profession, and the media, the gay community has taken the unusual step of forcing AIDS sufferers into the public eye. The tactic is surprising for several reasons. For one thing, it is natural to be reluctant to admit that one has contracted a contagious and incurable disease, especially a disease that carries the stigma of AIDS. Additionally, the attention, once gained, often involves the patient's identification as a homosexual, a categorization that still carries considerable risk in American society. Although the immediate aim of this bid for attention is to prolong life and assure treatment for those affected, a secondary effect will be to prevent any blocking out of reference to the AIDS epidemic from historical and literary records such as occurred in the previous century with the cholera epidemics.

Allowing the danger of AIDS to remain a private pestilence—that is, one the general public believes it may safely ignore because it is restricted to certain marginalized segments of the population—is what the gay community feels it cannot afford. For it is this attitude that has allowed responsible governmental agencies and some areas of the medical industry (especially the pharmaceutical companies) to slight the financial demands involved in AIDS research and patient care. Setting aside the desire for privacy that, with good reason, has been a primary concern for many homosexuals, the gay community has chosen to take a very public stand. Every act and demonstration, every book or publication on AIDS, thus gains a political significance. Gay activists purposely place the body of the diseased squarely within the public view and demand that it be gazed upon by the collective eye of government and populace. This tactic is a profound acknowledgment of visibility as the source of power in a democracy, a lesson learned perhaps from the struggle by American blacks for civil rights. (One need look no further than Ralph Ellison's *Invisible Man* [1952] for verification of this. Even earlier, Frederick Douglass observed in his *Narrative* that slaves in urban areas were treated differently from those on huge plantations because of the presence of neighbors as witnesses.)

Not surprisingly, contagion itself has paradoxically proven to be the greatest ally of those who struggle to achieve the necessary visibility for the disease and those who suffer from it. Once it became clear that AIDS is highly contagious and capable of moving from a minority to the general population, lobbying efforts began to bring results. Working against the fear and hysteria that contagion generates, while at the same time turning it to the best possible advantage, such groups as the Gay Men's Health Crisis have not only been in the forefront of the AIDS battle but have also become adroitly sensitive to changes in public attitudes, many of which they have themselves effected through education and publicity. Evidence that contagion is the spur to government spending comes from federal health officials who now defer requests from other health lobbyists by pointing out that AIDS is a contagious disease and therefore demands a larger share of available funds.[13]

= AIDS in Literature =

Fictional depictions of AIDS are not extensive; but if one looks beyond the categories of imaginative and critical writing, the list of works on the subject lengthens to include chronicles, memoirs, documentary films, and even a collective work of folk art. I have chosen to discuss those works that seem to me to reveal an honest understanding of the conditions faced by people most threatened by this epidemic, and that achieve, through superior writing, a universality of appeal.

The AIDS Reader: Social, Political, Ethical Issues (1991), edited by Nancy F. McKenzie, is an excellent anthology of essays and articles by leading activists from the viewpoints mentioned in the title; it contains no imaginative literature. The self-consciously literary writer Susan Sontag, in Aids and Its Metaphors (1988), concentrates on the metaphors and myths with which we literarily endow illness and disease. Ultimately her argument comes down to a dislike for both the older metaphors of disease fighting—such as "the war on cancer," which is now also frequently (and inappropriately) used to describe the approach to AIDS—and the newer metaphors having to do with virology that defuse and deflate the truly destructive action of viruses. Much of the literature on AIDS originating from the gay community is aimed at dispelling myths that have surrounded homosexuality, especially the sickness metaphor that is used in relation to it, and that the epidemic has reinforced. Not surprisingly, however, given the felt need to focus public attention on AIDS and its individual, human consequences, the visual element in literature has often predominated, perhaps at the expense of the text.

From the gay community have come such strong personal images as the televised AIDS diary of a San Francisco broadcast journalist, Paul Wynne, who until his death in the summer of 1990 appeared weekly on a program that chronicled the progress of his disease. Among the best literary efforts thus far are visually oriented works, such as the play by William Hoffman, As Is (1985), and another by Larry Kramer, The Normal Heart (1985), both discussed on page 139. Inherent in their dramatic form is the expectation of public viewing. The same is true of Terrence McNally's Andre's Mother, performed in 1989 as a television play and not now available in print. For a work done in the totally visual medium of television, *Andre's Mother* has a strange quality of invisibility woven into its plot, for Andre himself is never seen. Since the play deals with the consequences of Andre's death for his mother and his lover, his absence makes their loss almost palpable and effectively focuses attention on the body of the diseased. Unfortunately, the author's attempt to make Andre's memory a sainted one mars the play; it is an obvious overstatement that is designed to counter the feelings of antipathy a mass TV audience might feel toward such an unlikely hero. This effort to spiritualize AIDS patients is similar to the nineteenth-century view of tuberculosis victims and often finds its way into public discourse on the subject.

Two documentary films shown on television, *Positive* and *Silence Equals Death*, were produced by Rosa von Praunheim in 1990. The first examines the emotions of several individuals who have learned they are HIV-positive; the second takes a more wide-ranging approach to its subject and presents words and images created by a number of artists and writers, including the poet Allen Ginsberg, in response to the disease. Ginsberg exceeds the global perspective of some medical writers and sees the disease as a cosmic event with the planet Earth itself a victim. A 1991 documentary by Peter Adair entitled *Absolutely Positive* repeats the format offered by *Positive*; it adds little in the way of new knowledge but keeps the focus of television's commanding eye on the subject of AIDS.

The slogan "Silence equals death," which is used as the title of von Praunheim's documentary, is the slogan of ACT UP, the AIDS Coalition to Unleash Power, a group of extremely vocal—and visible—AIDS activists under the leadership of the group's founder, Larry Kramer. Kramer was a cofounder of New York City's Gay Men's Health Crisis; he was asked by that organization to resign his position because his approach was considered too confrontational and radical. Since its inception in 1987, ACT UP has engaged in confrontational politics of the most blatant and abrasive sort. To its credit, it has been responsible for changes in the medical system, the most important of which was persuading the government to make experimental drugs more accessible and at lowered costs; this change has meant the prolonging of hundreds of lives. ACT UP also continues to challenge individuals and institutions who refuse to take seriously the epidemic nature of AIDS and is now lobbying the CDC in an attempt to gain a revision of the federal description of AIDS to include those symptoms that mark the disease in women. One of the fastest growing groups of AIDS patients in the country, women cannot enter health insurance claims for their treatment because the official description of the disease as currently written excludes their symptoms.

For all its seriousness of purpose, ACT UP has never denied the strong element of street theater that is implied in its name and informs its public demonstrations. Many of these, especially those aimed at religious communities, seem like attempts to force acceptance of the gay community, and so

ACT UP is not without its critics. Part of the group's program is ongoing visual propaganda using posters and other graphics to tell the AIDS story. A collection of these graphics has been published as *AIDS Demo Graphics* (1990) which accentuates the high visibility sought by this organization for its cause and for AIDS sufferers.

Though so much of his life is now taken over by the political agenda of ACT UP, Larry Kramer is first of all a writer, and his *Reports from the holocaust* (1989) is a collection of articles that appeared originally in newspapers dating from the beginning of the epidemic in 1980. To this is added an essay, bearing the book's title, that is both a personal account and public document of life in a time of plague. It is not these articles, however, or the long and effective essay that have established Kramer as a writer of force and sensitivity, but rather his play *The Normal Heart*, produced in New York in 1985. Because it shares a theme and a coincidence of time with William Hoffman's play *As Is* (also produced in 1985), it is useful to consider them jointly.

= *As Is* and *The Normal Heart* =

Both *As Is* and *The Normal Heart* appeared in the year that the film star Rock Hudson died of AIDS; it was the year the disease "went public," one might say, in that Hudson's death brought the epidemic to the consciousness of many in the nation who had to that point remained ignorant of it. *As Is* is the story of two gay men, Richard and Saul, who at the play's opening are ending their relationship. Richard already has a new lover, and he also has AIDS. At the moment of his admission to Saul that he has contracted the disease the play moves into what becomes its most effective staging device—the use of multiple voices engaged in simultaneous conversations that fade in and out of each other but whose meanings mesh. The conversations involve family members, hospital personnel, friends, barroom pickups, and a hospice worker whose words begin and end the play, wrapping it in a cocoonlike warmth of mother-love for her dying patients. Effective though the multiple-voice device is, the characters never succeed in reaching each other or meshing, as do the structures of their fragmented conversations. Indeed, the chorus of fragments comes together thematically, much as in music, but the language generally seems at variance with the action.

Humor lightens the mood of the play and brings its own warmth but proves intrusive when it works against the plot. At the core of the play is Richard's desire to be accepted by his brother, who represents the straight world of married heterosexuality. In the play's most affecting moment, when the brothers embrace in Richard's hospital bed, the emotion is almost immediately turned to humor at the approach of a hospital orderly who misunderstands the scene and, in broken English, warns Richard that Saul is on his way to the room and will not be pleased to find him in the arms of another man. Although the intent may have been to prevent the play from turning maudlin, the haste with which the reconciliation between the brothers is brushed aside, and the blurring of genuine tenderness with sexual innuendo, suggests an uneasiness with male emotions that carries over into the play as a whole. The need for privacy, for covering genuine emotions with bantering and often self-mocking humor, cloaks the drama of the play—despite the chorus of voices that should serve as intermediaries between stage and audience—so that we feel ourselves intruders in this world, much as Richard's brother is. The temptation is to leave the world of Richard and Saul pretty much "as is," without feeling a sense of urgency about the plague that threatens it and us.

The Normal Heart depicts its author's involvement with the Gay Men's Health Crisis and his subsequent rejection by that group. The play explores both the public and private sides of its central character, Ned Weeks, as the AIDS epidemic impinges upon his life with increasing ferocity. As do many literary works dealing with homosexuality, the play reveals a deep longing for family, both the natural family of one's birth and the family relationships formed within a circle of friends. When he is asked to resign from the organization he has helped found, Ned Weeks once again experiences a feeling of having been rejected by his family, though his natural family has not so much rejected as ignored him in the hope that his "condition" will go away.

Ned is unable to forsake his public life, not even temporarily. In one scene he finds himself in the company of someone to whom he feels greatly attracted; he manages to turn the moment of mutual attraction into a protracted argument in which he draws an analogy between the Holocaust and the indifference of the public and the government to the AIDS crisis. Like its protagonist, the play is complex, brooding, and often powerful. It is complex in that it attempts a great deal (perhaps too much for the good of the play's unity): it explores not only political, social, and personal relationships but also individual reactions to the AIDS epidemic. Added to these elements is the love story of Ned and Felix, an affair made difficult by Ned's explosive anger and fierce defensiveness, and the medical story of AIDS, which comes to us from the perspective of a doctor whose practice is almost exclusively within the gay community and who is one of the first in New York City to recognize the epidemical proportions of the disease.

As in the Hoffman play, here too the crucial scene is one between brothers, Ned and his lawyer brother Ben. But Ned demands of Ben far more than the mere show of affection proffered in *As Is*. In his usual style, Ned confronts his brother, using as his premise the issue of sickness and health. This is the underlying issue of the play because, though he never admits it, the suspicion lingers in Ben's mind that Ned is sick, not with AIDS but with homosexuality, for which Ned has earlier received psychiatric "treatment." "Define it for me," Ned insists. "What do you mean by 'sick'? Sick unhealthy? Sick perverted? Sick I'll get over it? Sick to be locked up?"[14] He continues to badger Ben, trying to wring from him the declaration Ben cannot make: that he and Ned are the same, not one sick, one well. The argument ends with Ned resolving not to speak to Ben "until you accept me as your equal. Your healthy equal. Your brother!" (*Heart,* 71). In this one scene the play successfully combines the two halves of the protagonist's life, the private and the public, by making the issue of his personal health and his personal relationships— as in his relationship with his brother—a matter of public health, of healing the wound that separates into two halves the human family. When the reconciliation of the brothers occurs, the reconciliation of public and private health is implied, effectively saving the play's threatened unity.

=   Other Artistic Responses to AIDS   =
The Visual Prevails

Memoirs and memorials in various forms also help to focus attention on those dying of AIDS, and among these, Paul Monette's *Borrowed Time: An AIDS Memoir* (1988) is particularly affecting. Monette tells the story of the 19 months and 10 days of life that remained for his lover from the time a diagnosis was made in March 1985, and of the almost daily horrors the two men experienced during that time. In telling their story, the author reveals that he is himself HIV-positive; the added awareness of the teller's impending death intensifies the impact of this tale of death. The book reverses the familiar American survivor's tale (Ishmael in *Moby-Dick,* Arthur Mervyn in Brown's memoirs of the yellow fever epidemic, Frederick Douglass escaping his slavery, and Mary Rawlinson her captivity) and draws within its circle of immediate involvement the subject matter, the author, and the reader.

Paul Monette has also written two novels that deal with the impact of AIDS on the gay community, *Afterlife* (1990) and *Halfway Home* (1991). The first tells the story of three AIDS "widowers" who meet in the waiting room of the hospital where their lovers are dying. The book deals with the aftermath of the deaths in the lives of the survivors, and their coming to terms (or not) with loss and the knowledge of their own vulnerability. *Halfway Home* touches on a theme common in gay literature, the estrangement that develops between brothers when one is gay and the other is straight. In this story the relationship is further complicated by AIDS in the life of one, and white-collar crime in the life of the other. Humor and an exciting plot move the novel into areas not explored in the author's previous works, but the AIDS presence remains a constant, for it is, by force of circumstance, this author's primary subject.

Someone Was Here: Profiles in the AIDS Epidemic (1988) by George Whitmore is a book of interviews with people whose lives have been affected by the tragedy of AIDS. Though the stories they tell have been dramatized, the author notes in his preface that they are based on reality, a claim that appears to be well substantiated by the wealth of factual information in the work. Perhaps the most striking fact is one offered at the outset—that at the time the book begins, in February 1985, there were 8,495 diagnosed cases of AIDS in this country; when it ends, in February 1987, there were 31,036 cases.

The most unusual memorial to those who have died of AIDS has come not from the world of literature or drama but from handcraft—specifically, a type of needlework that is quintessentially American, quilting. The quilt is the product of the NAMES Project, a national endeavor begun in 1985 in a San Francisco storefront where seven volunteers began creating quilted panels commemorating victims of AIDS. The object was to design three-by-six-foot panels, each bearing the name of someone who had died of the disease, along with decorations illustrating that person's life. The panels were then sewn into larger quilt sections measuring twelve feet square. As the project grew other panels were solicited, and the response from across the nation was overwhelming.

In October 1987 the quilt was displayed in front of the U.S. Capitol in Washington, where it covered a space larger than two football fields. The following spring it traveled to 25 major American cities, returning to Washington in the fall of 1988. Panels continue to arrive from all the states, and the NAMES Project vows not to forsake the work. Cindy Ruskin tells the story of this highly unusual undertaking in *The Quilt: Stories from the NAMES Project* (1988), but it is the color reproductions that make this an exciting book. The individual panels are vibrant and highly decorative, funny and touching—and all presented in this most American of folk art forms.

Here again the visual element is predominant; the quilt creates a text that bears witness to those who have died of AIDS. Displaying it in Washington, D.C., not far from the memorial to the Vietnam War dead was a bold step that served to draw even more attention to the project. The contrast between the two memorials is equally bold, even if unintended. Both works list the names of the dead in a "lest we forget" gesture. The hard granite and forbidding color of the war memorial contrast sharply, however, with the softness and warmth of the quilt material embroidered over and appliquéd with colorful and fanciful designs. There is a certain daring, too, in using as a memorial for this disease a symbol associated with the bed, which in a post-Freudian age cannot ever lose its sexual connotations. Yet quilts also have a long relationship with American domesticity and have provided throughout our history opportunities for creativity and companionship as well as physical warmth. Of the quilting bee, the nineteenth-century communal gathering at which women worked together to create these home adornments, one book says, "Here women had the chance to form meaningful friendships in an atmosphere of Christian kindliness and charity."[15] Beyond its overt commemoration of the dead, the NAMES Project quilt suggests that these are qualities worth nurturing in all people.

A videotape in which the story of the quilt and its creation is told further intensifies the quilt's visual impact. The distribution in commercial video stores across the country of *Common Threads: Stories from the Quilt* (1989) deprives the idea of surveillance of its negative connotation by emphasizing the importance of the collective eye to an understanding of the human dimensions of the AIDS epidemic. The loss to the nation and the damage to the public health, or wholeness, represented by the deaths of so many AIDS victims cannot fail to make an impression on a nationwide audience.

The emphasis on the visual continues. During AIDS awareness days, held to heighten national consciousness of the gravity of the threat posed by the disease, paintings have been removed from museums and sculptures shrouded from view. The groups responsible for these efforts have denied any attempt to overtly link specific artists with the disease, but the effect is nonetheless a powerful reminder of the human and artistic loss that AIDS has wrought.

Perhaps the emphasis on the visual as a means of gaining personal and political power has worked to the detriment of literary productions, or perhaps too much creativity is being cut off too soon in this epidemic. Then, too, survivors may mourn best in more active ways, through political demonstrations, newspaper journalism, or even the time-honored art of needlework. Whatever the reason, there is not yet evidence that this epidemic will inspire a body of creative literature. Larry Kramer claims to be working on a long novel dealing with AIDS. "I feel like fate has placed me on the front lines of the battle," the playwright and activist comments, "and I'm here to report it in some sort of way. . . . Writers are often lucky enough to be given their subject matter, and if they're smart enough they recognize that it's there and grab it."[16] Kramer has revealed that he tested HIV-positive in October 1988 and openly admits his fear of not living to finish his novel.

In *Ground Zero* (1985), a book of essays about AIDS that largely mourns the passing of a time when one could heed the advice given to Milly Theale in James's *The Wings of the Dove*—to "live" without fear—Andrew Holleran explains the dearth of creative literature dealing with AIDS: "Someday—not just yet—there will be novels about all of this, but they will face the problem writing about it stumbles against now: how to include the individual stories, the astonishingly various ways in which people have behaved."[17]

While we await the novels, several short stories are available. One, "The Way We Live Now" by Susan Sontag, appeared in 1986 and thus predates the *Daedalus* study, yet its emphasis on living is the same, that is, "living *with* a disease."[18] Experimental in form, the story tells of one man's illness with an unnamed disease, which from all narrative indications is AIDS. The progress of the disease is described in a series of long paragraphs, each of which is a running commentary by the man's friends representing their varied reactions to and opinions on his health: "At first he was just losing weight, he felt only a little ill, Max said to Ellen, and he didn't call for an appointment with his doctor, according to Greg, because he was managing to keep on working at more or less the same rhythm, but he did stop smoking, Tanya pointed out, which suggests he was frightened, but also that he wanted, even more than he knew, to be healthy, or healthier, or maybe just to gain back a few pounds, said Orson, for he told her, Tanya went on, that he expected to be climbing the walls (isn't that what people say?) and found, to his surprise, that he didn't miss cigarettes at all and reveled in the sensation of his lungs' being ache-free for the first time in years" ("Way" 1168). The friends are alternately attentive, loving, quarrelsome, jealous of each other, and neglectful of the patient, as the term of his illness stretches out. While at one point one of them worries that their attentions are really a way of "trying to define ourselves more firmly and irrevocably as the well, those who aren't ill," they are, in fact, learning how to live with someone who is gravely ill, without the shame and avoidance that so often accompanies illness in our society. The story is, therefore, as much theirs as the unnamed patient's, and is as much concerned with the survival of hope in the midst of death as it is with the man's survival.

Of particular interest is the way in which Sontag attempts to reverse the "suffering victim" image symbolized by the all too familiar representations of a young Saint Sebastian pierced by arrows. The point is made that, according to the saint's legend, his suffering did not end in death; rather, when his body was being prepared for burial it was discovered that he was still alive, and his Christian friends nursed him back to health. As one of the friends in Sontag's story says, "[T]he difference between a story and a painting or photograph is that in a story you can write, He's still alive. But in a painting or a photo you can't show 'still.' You can just show him being alive" ("Way," 1179). The statement asserts literary over visual claims by properly emphasizing the precision of language in defining life, a precision echoed in the final statement by one of the friends on the condition of the sick man, "He's still alive" ("Way," 1179).

A collection of short stories by Allen Barnett, *The Body and Its Dangers* (1990), includes three stories that touch on AIDS and the ways people behave when confronted by it. The best of these (and of the collection) is "The *Times* as It Knows Us," a story of a group of gay men who have enjoyed good times together, and friendships, which the presence of disease among them has now brought to an end. Following the line of literary development predicted by Andrew Holleran, the plot is based on the various ways in which the friends respond to the epidemic. But what lifts the story above others in the collection is the premise on which the plot rests, the contrast between the private reality of AIDS and the public image of gay life in a time of epidemic, specifically as it is reported in a *New York Times* story for which one of the friends has agreed to be interviewed. The *Times* presents the men as superficial both in their mourning for the AIDS dead and in their concern for the AIDS-stricken; the general impression created by the newspaper story is that of Poe's "The Masque of the Red Death," with the gay community cast as the unheeding revelers.

Barnett's story is factually accurate in its reference to the *Time*'s long resistance to the use of the word *gay*, an editorial reluctance that pointed up the newspaper's negative attitude toward changing mores and seemed to explain its lack of interest in the spreading epidemic for the first half of the AIDS decade. The gay community that the *Times* story depicts is not the one that Barnett describes; among the latter group are some people who, like some in any given group, can handle the tragedy and others who cannot. One by one the circle of friends is affected by the disease, either directly or indirectly, and soon the *Times* story, which once had seemed so important to the men for its power to fashion a public image of gay life, shrinks into insignificance. As the narrator explains the inevitable withdrawal that occurs, "You let go of people, the living and the dead, and return to yourself, to your own resources, like a widower, a tourist alone in a foreign country."[19] Though the story points up the risk involved in seeking media attention, it does not, ultimately, deny the necessity of doing so.

═ From Image to Discourse ═

The tourist alone in a foreign country is often bereft of language and its compensations and is forced to rely on the visible signs by which he or she may know and be known. By these signs, of race, gender, age, class, and degree of affluence, we are known and categorized, just as we know and categorize others. So basic, so primary, is the perception of relative health that we seldom think to include it among these gross categories. Yet now, in the AIDS era, we know more clearly than ever the truth of Scott Fitzgerald's words, that there is no difference between people "so profound as the difference between the sick and the well." The desire to alter this notion of profound difference, as well as the images of the diseased, impels the gay community and others to words and acts that invite the gaze of public attention and that oppose the silence that equals death.

In that very slogan, "Silence equals death," adopted by many AIDS activists as a way of reminding themselves and others of their objective, there is an implied recourse to language and to public discourse as a defense against death.[20] But when visualized the slogan also suggests the mathematical calculation of a sum, in this case, the sum of those whose lives have been the cost of others' silence. Discussion, on a national level if possible, is the aim of the slogan, but in a society as visually oriented as ours it is imagery that stimulates discourse. Because of the deep-seated need of so many in our society to dissociate themselves from the AIDS patient, numerous images of these patients have been created that attempt to depict them as "other." The predominant image has been that of the sexual deviant, though it is now joined by that of the drug-addicted, yet another undesirable image (Gilman, 258–59). Counterimages involving artistry and imagination, such as those provided by the creators of the AIDS quilt, can become powerful tools toward delimiting the definition of "other," so that the attempt to isolate individuals stigmatized by AIDS is made more difficult. Errors of judgment can accompany this aim, however. Something like the softening of the grim reality of a tuberculosis death that occurred in the nineteenth century by associating it with the death of innocent children is beginning to surface in public images offered now of infants born with AIDS. Although this imagery may prove helpful in altering public perception of the AIDS patient, the sympathy thus aroused, like that for the TB sufferer who was thought to be spiritually refined by the disease, is misguided. In its blurring of reality the image deflects attention from the larger and truer picture of the horror of this disease, which is not confined to infants.

Though it has not yet received the wide attention its originators had hoped for, there is one image current in the gay community that has the symbolic potential of a Hawthorne emblem. The slogan "Silence equals death" is usually displayed graphically in white lettering set below a pink triangle. The pink triangle was the sign by which homosexuals were known during their captivity in Nazi concentration camps, and the image therefore arouses cognitive associations to that era and to the determination of Jews worldwide never to allow the camps to exist again. The symbol says much the same thing as Larry Kramer's equation of the AIDS epidemic with the Holocaust, but its visual impact is immediate and emotional, like the scarlet letter on Hester Prynne's breast. The reconciliation of opposing planes suggested by the scarlet A and the pink triangle, however, move both these emblems toward new mental associations. As used by the gay community, the triangle indicates this hoped-for reconciliation but goes beyond that hope to register the determination of a group now marginalized to insist on its right to define its collective identity and thus shape the comprehension of the greater society. As a means of expanding public perception the symbol can be highly effective since, especially in America, an image either speaks for itself or is spoken of by others, and one either defines the terms of discourse that arise from the image or allows others to articulate their perceptions of its meaning as truth.

Imaging, of the kind noted here, effectively reverses the posture of the body of the diseased, making it the subject rather than the object of the medical and societal gaze; imaging allows the subject-observer to articulate what is seen. Ultimately, imaging affirms a fundamental belief among Americans in the ability of individuals to act in concert, to empower themselves, and to undermine that power inherent in social institutions that to Foucault seemed both monolithic and invincible.

As I write, the AIDS epidemic is ten years old. There is talk every day of possible new treatments and medications, even of a vaccine that increases T-cell production in AIDS patients, boosting their ability to fight secondary, opportunistic infections and thus prolong their lives. The annual international conference on AIDS (with U.S. Public Health Service representation drastically reduced by the federal government) met in 1991 amid speculation that the coming year would see large-scale efficacy trials for a variety of vaccines. But the prospect raises a plethora of potential horrors: such testing requires that humans be exposed to the live virus, and if the experiment fails they will die. Even should it succeed, those inoculated will forever after test HIV-positive, a status that, in the present atmosphere of American society, could subject them to loss of employment, friends, and much that gives meaning to life. Fear of either outcome could inhibit medical advances and prolong the epidemic.

While the medical community continues its struggle and government agencies continue theirs, the number of individuals affected by the disease continues to rise: more than 175,000 Americans have developed AIDS, and 109,000 have died of it; an estimated one million more are infected with the AIDS virus. When one also considers the effect of each of these illnesses and deaths on those close to the patients, the sheer number of people involved is staggering. It may be that the weight of these statistics bears so heavily on the creative minds of the nation's literary community that the production of imaginative literature dealing with the subject remains limited. Or it may be that with a decade of living with AIDS behind us we are just beginning to come to terms with the disease, literally and literarily. Thus far there have been no literary works dealing with the epidemic within the heterosexual community; as the disease spreads into that population these may appear. The critic tends to hope that literature will arise from any situation, but it may be that for many writers the present epidemic is too grim to allow direct literary treatment, and that future critics and scholars will detect its presence as a subtext in works ostensibly dealing with other subjects. If such should prove to be the case, scholars will require texts that overtly detail the AIDS experience against which to test their speculations. They will be well served by those discussed in this chapter.

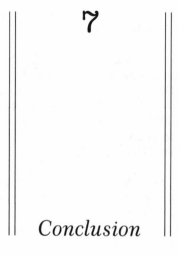

7

Conclusion

THE UNITED STATES OF AMERICA IS 200 YEARS REMOVED from an epidemic that threatened the very continuance of the nation, yet it finds itself still having to cope with epidemical disease. Far from being immune to such evils, the New World repeatedly has been the site of epidemics; at present, while North America is engulfed in the AIDS outbreak, South America is seeing the return of cholera, the first occurrence of the disease in the New World in this century. No matter what advantage is gained by modern medicine, it seems that epidemics will remain a part of human history. At best Americans can only hope to benefit from the steady advance of medical knowledge, which has brought vaccines and cures for most epidemical diseases. They can benefit as well from an understanding of their historical responses to epidemics and be guided by the best of these.

In chapter 1, I set forth three responses to epidemics revealed by my reading of American historical and literary sources: (1) the panic response, which seeks solely to identify and isolate the source of infection; (2) the denial response, which refuses to acknowledge the presence of an epidemic;

and (3) the rational, scientific response, which seeks to identify the source of infection and to treat both the disease and its cause. Evidence drawn from the historical and literary record indicates that in most instances of epidemic in America a response of any kind is slow to formulate. This is not surprising given American reluctance to admit the presence of pestilence, pollution, or whatever other word is conjured up by the idea of epidemic. Largely because of this reluctance, whatever response is made often evolves, so that an initial denial may eventually change into a panic or a rational response. As the discussion of the AIDS epidemic reveals, America is currently in the process of moving from a posture of denial of the extent of the epidemic toward the rational approach of educating about the disease in the hope of reducing the number of new cases. An earlier tendency toward a panic response has been alleviated, for the most part, by this same rational approach, and the persistence of some affected groups in turning attention on themselves has prevented the use of authoritative power to isolate them.

Clearly the greatest potential for a panic reaction in America existed during the yellow fever epidemics of the 1790s, when the new nation felt itself vulnerable on all sides. Panic, denial, and reason all combined in a confusion of responses that reflected the general confusion created by the fever. The literary record of the yellow fever epidemics enhances the historical to a degree unmatched by other epidemics. The imaginative depictions of yellow fever tend toward a romantic emphasis on the erroneous speculation that surrounded it; literature pertaining to tuberculosis, on the other hand, follows the rational approach of science by attempting to understand the underlying connections between the disease and the society in which it appeared. These approaches correspond to the period's romantic literature, which for the most part veiled its subject behind other concerns, and to the realistic literature that followed.

Even in the most obvious instance of denial, the three cholera epidemics of the nineteenth century, an official response eventually evolved that, reasonably, recognized the need for clean drinking water and better sanitation. And in the 1721 smallpox epidemic in Boston it was the scientism of Cotton Mather and others like him that dispelled not only the disease but the possibility of a panic reaction such as that which earlier had incited the witch trials. In Hawthorne's tale of this epidemic the author appears to have had a problem balancing this rationality, and the spirit of revolution it provoked, with the theological import of the Puritan settlement in America. Hawthorne's treatment of the subject is important because of his preeminence among nineteenth-century American writers and because of his historical and cultural perspective. What we learn from him tells us a great deal about Americans in general, of his time and ours. Hawthorne was actually too close, both temporally and geographically, to the smallpox epidemic to recognize it for what it was—a turning away from the Puritan medievalism of the seventeenth century and toward the modern age. Yet by linking the epidemic with the breakdown of British rule that was to come, he reenacted the part of the physician in the modern world who deals with epidemics by seeking the source in the surrounding environment. Although the tale itself is undeniably the stuff of romanticism, in which too often the peering medical eye violates by its surveillance the sanctity of human life, the reenactment is not. Instead, it exhibits the medical consciousness of a new age that hoped by observation of the processes of life, death, and disease to learn the connections between them. Whether he was comfortable with the new position or not, Hawthorne, like Cotton Mather, had already made the shift toward the modern world and was ready to think of epidemics in human as well as divine terms.

CHRONOLOGY

1714   John Woodward, London physician, publishes account of smallpox inoculations in Constantinople.

1718   Lady Mary Wortley Montagu, "Inoculation Against Smallpox"; describes procedure as witnessed in Constantinople.

1721   Smallpox epidemic strikes Boston, the worst in city history. Urged by Cotton Mather, inoculations begin in colonies; inoculations introduced later the same year in England. James Franklin begins publishing the *New-England Courant* with brother Benjamin as apprentice.

1722   Benjamin Franklin writes "Silence Dogood" letters.

1749   First three volumes of *Histoire naturelle* by George Louis Leclerc, Comte de Buffon, are published; he sees nature as deformed in New World.

1785   Thomas Jefferson's *Notes on the State of Virginia*, which refutes Buffon, is published.

1789   Revolution in France.

1790   Philadelphia is named capital of the United States.

1791   New York Hospital opens.

1793   The Reign of Terror begins in France. Yellow fever hits Philadelphia, the worst epidemic in history for any U.S. city; fever returns almost every year until the end of the century and also appears in New York City. Elihu Hubbard Smith establishes his medical practice in New York City.

1795   First medical journal in America, *The Medical Repository*, edited by Smith and Dr. Samuel Latham Mitchill, is founded.

1796   Dr. Edward Jenner introduces cowpox vaccination into England as a smallpox preventative. *Collection of Papers on the Subject of Bilious Fevers Prevalent in the U.S. for a Few Years Past* (edited by Noah Webster, Jr.), containing Smith's letters on yellow fever, is published.

1798   Congress passes Alien and Sedition Acts. Public Health Service created by Congress to prevent outbreak of epidemics. Smith dies of yellow fever in New York City; his friend Charles Brockden Brown survives.

1799   Brown's *Ormond, Arthur Mervyn, Part I*, and *Edgar Huntly* are published.

1800   Brown's *Arthur Mervyn, Part II*, is published.

1804   C. F. Volney, *A View of the Soil and Climate of the United States of America*, translated by Brown, is published.

1826   Ralph Waldo Emerson travels south to recover from tuberculosis.

1831   Emerson's wife Ellen dies from tuberculosis.

1832   The first cholera epidemic in the New World strikes New York City.

1835   Edgar Allan Poe's "King Pest: A Tale Containing an Allegory," a story about the bubonic plague in fourteenth-century London, is published.

1836   Emerson's *Nature* is published.

1838   Nathaniel Hawthorne's "Lady Eleanore's Mantle," based on the 1721 smallpox epidemic in Boston, is published.

1842   Poe's "Masque of the Red Death," a tale of pestilence, is published.

1843   Oliver Wendell Holmes presents his paper "Contagiousness of Puerperal Fever" in Boston, anticipating Semmelweis in Vienna (1847).

1845–1847   Henry David Thoreau lives at Walden Pond.

1847   Karl Marx's *The Communist Manifesto* is published. The American Medical Association is founded.

1849	Second cholera epidemic strikes New York City.
1852	Harriet Beecher Stowe's *Uncle Tom's Cabin* is published; she establishes the image of the tubercular child, reinforced by Louisa May Alcott's *Little Women* (1868).
1854	Thoreau's *Walden* is published.
1862	Thoreau dies of tuberculosis.
1866	Third cholera epidemic strikes New York City.
1879	Henry James's *Daisy Miller*, in which the heroine dies of malaria, is published.
1881	James's *The Portrait of a Lady*, which contains a principal character who dies of tuberculosis, is published.
1882	Dr. Robert Koch in Germany discovers the germ responsible for tuberculosis.
1884	Sanitorium at Saranac Lake, New York, opens. Antituberculosis campaign begins.
1895	Discovery of X-ray by Wilhelm Roentgen in Germany aids in early diagnosis of tuberculosis.
1900	Walter Reed is named head of U.S. Army Yellow Fever Commission; begins experiments (with associates James Carroll, Jesse Lazear, and Aristides Agramonte) that prove the theory of mosquito transmission of yellow fever.
1902	James's *The Wings of the Dove*, in which the heroine dies of tuberculosis, is published.
1904	National Association for Study and Prevention of Tuberculosis is founded.
1904–1906	Col. William C. Gorgas, applying techniques worked out by Reed, eliminates yellow fever from Panama Canal Zone.
1905	Willa Cather's "Paul's Case," a short story with a tubercular protagonist, is published.
1912	Eugene O'Neill contracts tuberculosis.
1914	World War I begins in Europe. The Panama Canal opens.
1917	The United States enters World War I.
1918–1919	Worldwide influenza epidemic kills an estimated 600,000 in the United States.
1919	O'Neill's *The Straw*, a play using his experiences as a patient in a TB sanitorium, is produced.
1920	O'Neill's *Beyond the Horizon*, in which the hero contracts TB, is produced; play will be awarded 1921 Pulitzer Prize.
1924	Thomas Mann's *The Magic Mountain* is published.
1929	Penicillin discovered by Dr. Alexander Fleming in London;

the drug will be used to treat syphilis. Thomas Wolfe's *Look Homeward, Angel* is published.

1932–1972   The PHS experiments on syphilitic black male sharecroppers in Tuskegee, Alabama, without their knowledge.

1938   Wolfe dies of tuberculosis of the brain.

1939   Katherine Anne Porter's "Pale Horse, Pale Rider," a short story based on the author's experience as an influenza victim in the 1918 epidemic, is published.

1950   Elia Kazan's film *Panic in the Streets* is released.

1952   Isoniazid is introduced as a treatment for tuberculosis. Epidemic of poliomyelitis strikes 60,000 in the United States.

1954   Dr. Jonas Salk develops injectable polio vaccine.

1956   O'Neill's *Long Day's Journey into Night*, a play (written in 1940) telling the story of how the author contracted tuberculosis, is produced.

1976   A mysterious flu afflicts American Legion conventioneers in Philadelphia, killing 29; subsequently named Legionnaires' disease. An epidemic of swine flu inspires a national program of inoculation.

1980–1981   First cases of pneumocystis carinii pneumonia appear in California and New York; the Centers for Disease Control forms a task force to study this and related cases of Kaposi's sarcoma and names the disease gay-related infectious disease.

1982   First international symposium on the epidemic of the disease now called acquired immune deficiency syndrome (AIDS) is held in July.

1983   The PHS releases guidelines for blood donations in recognition of new awareness that the disease is blood-transmissible; World Health Organization holds first meeting on AIDS epidemic.

1986   U. S. Surgeon General Dr. C. Everett Koop issues "Report on Acquired Immune Deficiency," advocating widespread education on the disease.

1987   AZT, a drug used to delay onset of AIDS symptoms in HIV-positive patients, is discovered.

1991   More than 100,000 Americans have died of AIDS, and an estimated one million are infected with the virus.

NOTES AND REFERENCES

Introduction

1. Jeremy Bentham, *A Fragment on Government and An Introduction to the Principles of Morals and Legislation*, ed. W. Harrison (Oxford: Basil Blackwell, 1970), 3.

2. Ralph Waldo Emerson, *Nature* [1836], in *Selections from Ralph Waldo Emerson: An Organic Anthology*, ed. Stephen E. Whicher (Boston: Houghton Mifflin, 1957), 24; hereafter cited in the text as Whicher.

3. Michel Foucault, *The Birth of the Clinic: An Archaeology of Medical Perception*, tr. A. M. Sheridan Smith (New York: Random House, 1973), 29, hereafter cited in the text.

4. Oliver Wendell Holmes, "The Contagiousness of Puerperal Fever," in *Medical Essays* (Boston: Houghton Mifflin, 1883), 169.

5. Quoted in Wilson G. Smilie, *Public Health: Its Promise for the Future* (New York: Arno, 1976), 159.

6. John T. Morse, Jr., ed., *The Life and Letters of Oliver Wendell Holmes*, vol. 1 (Boston: Houghton Mifflin, 1896), 93–94.

7. Richard Harrison Shryock, *Medicine and Society in America, 1660–1860* (Ithaca, N.Y.: Cornell University Press, 1960), 67, hereafter cited in the text.

8. Quoted in Michel Ciment, *Kazan on Kazan* (New York: Viking, 1975), 63.

9. Quoted in Alfred W. Crosby, *America's Forgotten Pandemic: The Influenza of 1918* (Cambridge, Mass.: Harvard University Press, 1989), 53, hereafter cited in the text.

10. Katherine Anne Porter, "Pale Horse, Pale Rider," in *Pale Horse, Pale Rider: Three Short Novels* (New York: Harcourt, Brace, 1936), 181, hereafter cited in the text as "Horse."

11. Joan Givner, *Katherine Anne Porter: A Life* (New York: Simon and Schuster, 1982), 127.

12. Horton Foote, *Courtship, Valentine's Day, 1918* (New York: Grove Press, 1987), 131.

13. "Once Again, a Man with a Mission," *New York Times Magazine*, 25 November 1990, 57–61.

The Pathology of Revolution

1. William H. McNeill, *Plagues and People* (Garden City, N.Y.: Doubleday, 1976), 207, hereafter cited in the text.

2. Thomas Babington Macaulay, *The History of England from the Accession of James II* (Philadelphia: 1887), 4:575.

3. Kenneth Silverman, *The Life and Times of Cotton Mather* (New York: Columbia University Press, 1985), 98, hereafter cited in the text as Silverman.

4. John Duffy, *Epidemics in Colonial America* (Baton Rouge: Louisiana State University Press, 1953), 51.

5. James A. Sappenfield, *A Sweet Instruction: Franklin's Journalism as a Literary Apprenticeship* (Carbondale: Southern Illinois University Press, 1973), 29–46, details each of the letters.

6. Perry Miller, *The New England Mind: From Colony to Province* (Boston: Beacon, 1953), 349, hereafter cited in the text.

7. Sacvan Bercovitch, *The American Jeremiad* (Madison: University of Wisconsin Press, 1978), xi.

8. Nathaniel Hawthorne, "Lady Eleanore's Mantle," in *Twice-Told Tales* [1837] (Columbus: Ohio State University Press, 1974), 273, hereafter cited in the text as "Mantle."

9. Sander L. Gilman, *Disease and Representation: Images of Illness from Madness to AIDS* (Ithaca, N.Y.: Cornell University Press, 1988), 256, hereafter cited in the text.

10. Sheldon W. Liebman, "Ambiguity in 'Lady Eleanore's Mantle,' " *Emerson Society Quarterly* 58 (1970): 97–101, hereafter cited in the text.

11. Michael Colacurcio, *The Province of Piety* (Cambridge, Massachusetts: Harvard University Press, 1984), 436–37, hereafter cited in the text.

The American Plague

1. George Washington Cable, *The Creoles of Louisiana* (New York: Scribner's, 1884), 298–99.

2. George Washington Cable, *The Grandissimes* (New York: Hill and Wang, 1957), 8.

3. Paul de Kruif, *Microbe Hunters* (New York: Blue Ribbon Books, 1926), 328–29.

4. Sidney Howard White, *Sidney Howard* (Boston: Twayne, 1977), 109.

5. Ian Cameron, *The Impossible Dream: The Building of the Panama Canal* (New York: Morrow, 1972), 134.

6. Quoted in John Edgar Wideman, "Fever," in *Fever: Twelve Stories* (New York: Henry Holt, 1989), 127, hereafter cited in the text as "Fever."

7. Elihu Hubbard Smith, letter to Charles Brockden Brown, 7 May 1796, in *The Diary of Elihu Hubbard Smith, 1771–1798*, ed. James E. Cronin (Philadelphia: American Philosophical Society, 1973), 164, hereafter cited in the text as Cronin.

8. Fred Lewis Pattee, ed., *The Poems of Philip Freneau*, vol. 1 (Princeton, N.J.: Princeton University Library, 1907), 81, hereafter cited in the text as Pattee.

9. George Louis Leclerc, Comte de Buffon, *Histoire naturelle*, 44 vols. (London, 1749–1804); Abbe Raynal, *Histoire philosophique et politique des éstablissements et du commerce des Européens dans les deux Indes* (London, 1770); Pehr Kalm, *Travels into North America* (London, 1753–61); and Corneille De Pauw, *Recherches philosophiques sur les Americains*, 2 vols. (Berlin, 1768), hereafter cited in the text as *Recherches*.

10. C. F. Volney, *Tableau du climat et sol des Etats Unis* (A View of the Soil and Climate of the United States of America), trans. Charles Brockden Brown (New York: Hafner Publishing, 1968), 249n, hereafter cited in the text as *View*.

11. John C. Miller, *Crisis in Freedom: The Alien and Sedition Acts* (Boston: Little, Brown, 1951), presents the full history of these laws.

12. E. H. Smith, "The Plague of Athens," *The Medical Repository*, vol. 1, no. 1, 29.

13. William Marshall, *A Theological Dissertation on the Propriety of Removing from the Seat of the Pestilence* (Philadelphia 1799) (unnumbered).

14. John K. Alexander, "Poverty, Fear, and Continuity: An Analysis of the Poor in Late Eighteenth-Century Philadelphia," in *The Peoples of Philadelphia*, ed. Alan F. Davis and Mark H. Haller, 13–35 (Philadelphia: Temple University Press, 1973).

15. Charles Brockden Brown, *Ormond, or, The Secret Witness* [1799] (Kent, Ohio: Kent State University Press, 1982), 36.

16. Charles Brockden Brown, *Arthur Mervyn, or, Memoirs of the Year 1793* [1799–1800] (Kent, Ohio: Kent State University Press, 1977), 144, hereafter cited in the text as *Mervyn*.

17. *The Present State of Medical Learning in the City of New York* [1797], quoted in Marcia E. Bailey, *A Lesser Hartford Wit: Dr. Elihu Hubbard Smith* (Orono, Maine: The University Press, 1928), 93.

18. Elihu Hubbard Smith, *A Collection of Papers on the Subject of Bilious Fevers Prevalent in the U.S. for a Few Years Past*, ed. Noah Webster, Jr. (New York, 1796), 248, hereafter cited in the text as *Papers*.

19. David R. Shumway, *Michel Foucault* (Boston: Twayne, 1989), 50.

20. Lloyd G. Stevenson, "Putting Disease on the Map: The Early Use of Spot Maps in the Study of Yellow Fever," *Journal of the History of Medicine and Allied Sciences* (vol. 20, 1965): 226–61. Seaman's map appears in *The Medical Repository* 1 (February 1798), facing p. 316.

21. Charles Brockden Brown to James Brown, 18 September 1798, in

William Dunlap, *The Life of Charles Brockden Brown*, vol. 2 (Philadelphia, 1815), 9–10.

22. Charles Brockden Brown, *Edgar Huntly, or, Memoirs of a Sleep-Walker* [1799], ed. Sydney J. Krause and S. W. Reid (Kent, Ohio: Kent State University Press, 1984), 3, hereafter cited in the text as *Huntly*.

23. Alexis de Tocqueville [1835], *Democracy in America*, ed. Richard D. Heffner (New York: New American Library, 1956), 177.

The Disease of Poverty

1. "Revenge and Requital: A Tale of a Murderer Escaped," *Democratic Review* [July-August 1845], reprinted in revised form as "One Wicked Impulse!" in *Walt Whitman: The Early Poems and the Fiction*, ed. Thomas L. Brasher, 309–18 (New York: New York University Press, 1963), 316.

2. Walt Whitman, "Song of Myself," in *Leaves of Grass* [1855], Comprehensive Reader's Edition, ed. Harold W. Blodgett and Sculley Bradley (New York: W. W. Norton, 1965), 72.

3. Charles E. Rosenberg, *The Cholera Years: The United States in 1832, 1849, and 1866* (Chicago: University of Chicago Press, 1962), hereafter cited in the text.

4. John Duffy, *A History of Public Health in New York City, 1625–1866* (New York: Russell Sage Foundation, 1968), 271.

5. This development is detailed by David J. Rothman, *The Discovery of the Asylum: Social Order and Disorder in the New Republic* (Boston: Little, Brown, 1971), hereafter cited in the text.

6. Geoffrey Marks and William K. Beatty, *Epidemics* (New York: Scribner's, 1976), 195.

7. Sarah Webster Goodwin, "Poe's 'Masque of the Red Death' and the 'Dance of Death,'" in *Medievalism in American Culture: Special Studies*, ed. Bernard Rosenthal and Paul E. Szarmach, 17–28 (Binghamton: State University of New York, CEMERS, 1987).

8. Edward H. Davidson, ed., *Selected Writings of Edgar Allan Poe* (Boston: Houghton Mifflin, 1956), 180.

The Disease That "Rides Mankind"

1. Susan Sontag, *Illness as Metaphor* (New York: Farrar, Straus and Giroux, 1978), 14, hereafter cited in the text.

2. Henry David Thoreau, *Walden, or Life in the Woods*, in *The Writings of Henry David Thoreau* [1906], vol. 2 (New York: AMS Press, 1968), 102, hereafter cited in the text as *Walden*.

3. Quoted in Elizabeth Nowell, *Thomas Wolfe: A Biography* (Garden City, N.Y.: Doubleday, 1960), 56, hereafter cited in the text.

4. Thomas Wolfe, *Look Homeward, Angel* (New York: Scribner's/Modern Library, 1929), 557.

5. Quoted in Ralph L. Rusk, *The Life of Ralph Waldo Emerson* (New York: Charles Scribner's Sons, 1949), 120, hereafter cited in the text.

6. Louisa May Alcott, *Little Women* [1868–69] (New York: World, 1969), 414.

7. Harriet Beecher Stowe, *Uncle Tom's Cabin, or, Life among the Lowly* [1852] (New York: Penguin American Library, 1981), 424.

8. Walter Harding, *The Days of Henry Thoreau: A Biography* [New York: Knopf, 1965] (New York: Dover, 1982), 442, hereafter cited in the text.

9. Walter Harding and Carl Bode, eds., *The Correspondence of Henry David Thoreau* (New York: New York University Press, 1958), 609.

10. T. J. Jackson Lears, *No Place of Grace: Antimodernism and the Transformation of American Culture, 1880–1920* (New York: Pantheon, 1981).

11. John Weiss, ed., *Life and Correspondence of Theodore Parker*, vol. 2 [1864] (Freeport, N.Y.: Books for Libraries Press, 1969), 513–15.

12. E. Richard Brown, *Rockefeller's Medicine Men: Medicine and Capitalism in America* (Berkeley: University of California Press, 1979), 70–75, hereafter cited in the text.

13. John Shaw Billings, "Jurisprudence of Hygiene" (1879), quoted in Smillie, *Public Health*, 1.

14. Mark Caldwell, *The Last Crusade: The War on Consumption, 1862–1954* (New York: Atheneum, 1988), 64.

15. Willa Cather, "Paul's Case," in *Willa Cather's Collected Short Fiction, 1892–1912*, ed. Virginia Faulkner (Lincoln: University of Nebraska Press, 1965), 253, hereafter cited in the text as "Case."

16. Christina Rossetti, "Goblin Market," *Norton Anthology of English Literature*, vol. 2, ed. M. H. Abrams (New York: W. W. Norton, 1979), 1524.

17. Arthur and Barbara Gelb, *O'Neill* (New York: Harper & Row, 1962), 231, hereafter cited in the text.

18. Talcott Parsons, "Health and Illness in the Light of American Values," in *Concepts of Health and Disease: Interdisciplinary Perspectives*, ed. Arthur L. Caplan, et al. (Reading, Massachusetts: Addison-Wesley, 1981), 57–81.

19. Jan W. Dietrickson, *The Image of Money in the American Novel of the Gilded Age* (New York: Humanities Press, 1969), 155.

20. Henry James, *The Wings of a Dove*, New York Edition (New York: Scribner's, 1909), v, hereafter cited in the text as *Wings*.

21. Leon Edel, ed., *Henry James Letters, 1843–1875*, vol. 1 (Cambridge, Mass.: Harvard University Press, 1974), 223–24, hereafter cited in the text as *Letters*.

22. Jean Strouse, *Alice James: A Biography* (Boston: Houghton Mifflin, 1980), 111.

23. Virginia C. Fowler, *Henry James' American Girl: The Embroidery on the Canvas* (Madison: University of Wisconsin Press, 1984), 86.

24. F. Scott Fitzgerald, *The Great Gatsby* (New York: Scribner's, 1925), 82.

25. William H. Gilman and J. E. Parsons, eds., *Journals and Miscellaneous Notebooks of Ralph Waldo Emerson*, vol. 8 (Cambridge, Mass.: Harvard University Press, 1970), 375.

A Private Pestilence

1. Panos Dossier, *AIDS and the Third World* (Philadelphia: New Society, 1989), 118–20.

2. Editors' introduction, "Living with AIDS," *Daedalus* 118, no. 3 (Summer 1989): xv.

3. Randy Shilts, *And the Band Played on: Politics, People, and the AIDS Epidemic* (New York: St. Martin's, 1987), xxii, hereafter cited in the text.

4. For the facts on AIDS I am indebted to Margaret A. Hamburg and Anthony S. Fauci, "AIDS: The Challenge to Biomedical Research," *Daedalus* 118, no. 2 (1989): 19–39.

5. "Puzzle of Sailor's Death Solved after 31 Years: The Answer Is AIDS," *New York Times*, 24 July 1990.

6. Lawrence K. Altman, M.D., "Gains Cited on AIDS, but Urgency Remains," *New York Times*, 25 June 1991.

7. "Doctors and Nurses Support AIDS Testing, Survey Shows," *New York Times*, 15 June 1991.

8. Ronald Bayer, "AIDS, Privacy, and Responsibility," *Daedalus* 118, no. 3 (1989): 79–99.

9. Sandra Panem, *The AIDS Bureaucracy* (Cambridge, Mass.: Harvard University Press, 1988), 68.

10. James H. Jones, *Bad Blood: The Tuskegee Syphilis Experiment* (New York: Free Press, 1981), 48. Though it remains unpublished a play written by David Feldshuh, M.D., *Miss Evers's Boys*, deals with the study. It was produced in Baltimore in December 1989.

11. "Talk of Government Being out to Get Blacks Falls on More Attentive Ears," *New York Times*, 29 October 1990.

12. Nicholas A. Christakis, "Responding to a Pandemic: International Interests in AIDS Control," *Daedalus* 118, no. 2 (1989): 113–34.

13. "Turning Disease Into Political Cause," *New York Times*, 7 January 1991.

14. Larry Kramer, *The Normal Heart* (New York: New American Library, 1985), 69, hereafter cited in the text as *Heart*.

15. Susan Burroughs Swan, *Plain and Fancy: American Women and Their Needlework, 1700–1850* (New York: Holt, Rinehart & Winston, 1977), 209.

16. Quoted in B. D. Colen, "AIDS: The First Decade," *Newsday*, 4 June 1991.

17. Andrew Holleran, *Ground Zero* (New York: Morrow, 1985), 27.

18. Susan Sontag, "The Way We Live Now," *The Houghton Mifflin Anthology of Short Fiction*, ed. Patricia Hampl (Boston: Houghton Mifflin, 1989), 1173; hereafter cited in the text as "Way."

19. Allen Barnett, *The Body and Its Dangers* (New York: St. Martin's, 1990), 116.

20. Lee Edelman, "Politics, Literary Theory, and AIDS," *South Atlantic Quarterly* 88, no. 1 (Winter 1989): 301–17.

BIBLIOGRAPHY

General

Ciment, Michel. *Kazan on Kazan*. New York: Viking, 1975.

Fitzgerald, F. Scott. *The Great Gatsby*. New York: Scribner's, 1925.

Foucault, Michel. *The Birth of the Clinic: An Archaeology of Medical Perception*. Translated by A. M. Sheridan Smith. New York: Random House, 1973.

————. Discipline and Punish: The Birth of the Prison. Translated by Alan Sheridan. New York: Pantheon, 1977.

Gilman, Sander L. *Disease and Representation: Images of Illness from Madness to AIDS*. Ithaca, N.Y.: Cornell University Press, 1988.

Holmes, Oliver Wendell. "The Contagiousness of Puerperal Fever." In *Medical Essays*. Boston: Houghton Mifflin, 1883.

————. *The Life and Letters of Oliver Wendell Holmes*, 2 vols. Edited by John T. Morse, Jr. Boston: Houghton Mifflin, 1896.

King, Lester S. *Transformations in American Medicine from Benjamin Rush to William Osler*. Baltimore: Johns Hopkins University Press, 1991.

Marks, Geoffrey, and William K. Beatty. *Epidemics*. New York: Scribner's, 1976.

McNeill, William H. *Plagues and People*. Garden City, N.Y.: Doubleday, 1976.

Pauly, Thomas H. *An American Odyssey: Elia Kazan and American Culture*. Philadelphia: Temple University Press, 1983.

Rothman, David J. *The Discovery of the Asylum: Social Order and Disorder in the New Republic.* Boston: Little, Brown, 1971.
Shryock, Richard Harrison. *Medicine and Society in America, 1660–1860.* Ithaca, N.Y.: Cornell University Press, 1960.
Shumway, David R. *Michel Foucault.* Boston: Twayne, 1989.
Smillie, Wilson G. *Public Health: Its Promise for the Future.* New York: Arno, 1976.
Sontag, Susan. *Illness as Metaphor.* New York: Farrar, Straus and Giroux, 1978.
Swan, Susan Burroughs. *Plain and Fancy: American Women and Their Needlework, 1700–1850.* New York: Holt, Rinehart & Winston, 1977.
Tocqueville, Alexis de. *Democracy in America* [1835]. Edited by Richard D. Heffner. New York: New American Library, 1956.
Winslow, Charles-Edward Amory. *Man and Epidemics.* Princeton, N.J.: Princeton University Press, 1952.

AIDS

ACT UP. AIDS Demo Graphics. Seattle: Bay Press, 1990.
Barnett, Allen. *The Body and Its Dangers.* New York: St. Martin's, 1990.
Bayer, Ronald. "AIDS, Privacy, and Responsibility." *Daedalus* 118, no. 3 (1989): 79–99.
Cahill, Kevin M., ed. *The AIDS Epidemic.* New York: St. Martin's, 1983.
Christakis, Nicholas A. "Responding to a Pandemic: International Interests in AIDS Control." *Daedalus* 118, no. 2 (1989): 113–34.
Dossier, Panos. AIDS and the Third World. Philadelphia: New Society, 1989.
Edelman, Lee. "Politics, Literary Theory, and AIDS." *South Atlantic Quarterly* 88, no. 1 (Winter 1989): 301–17.
Feldman, Douglas A. *Culture and AIDS.* Westport, Conn.: Praeger, 1990.
Gallo, Robert. *Virus Hunting: AIDS, Cancer, and the Human Retrovirus: A Story of Scientific Discovery.* New York: Basic, 1991.
Gilman. *Disease and Representation.* See under General.
Hamburg, Margaret A., and Anthony S. Fauci. "AIDS: The Challenge to Biomedical Research." *Daedalus* 118, no. 2 (1989): 19–39.
Hoffman, William. *As Is.* New York: Random House, 1985.
Holleran, Andrew. *Ground Zero.* New York: Morrow, 1985.
Kinsella, James. *Covering the Plague: AIDS and the American Media.* New Brunswick, N.J.: Rutgers University Press, 1989.
Kramer, Larry. *The Normal Heart.* New York: New American Library, 1985.
———. *Reports from the holocaust.* New York: St. Martin's, 1989.
Living with AIDS. Daedalus 118, nos. 2 and 3 (1989).
McKenzie, Nancy F., ed. *The AIDS Reader: Social, Political, Ethical Issues.* New York: New American Library, 1991.
Monette, Paul. *Borrowed Time: An AIDS Memoir.* New York: Avon, 1988.
———. *Afterlife.* New York: Avon, 1990.
———. *Halfway Home.* New York: Avon, 1991.
Panem, Sandra. *The AIDS Bureaucracy.* Cambridge, Mass.: Harvard University Press, 1988.
Rodetsky, Peter. *The Invisible Invaders: The Story of the Emerging Age of Viruses.* Boston: Little, Brown, 1991.

Ruskin, Cindy. *The Quilt: Stories from the NAMES Project*. New York: Pocket, 1988.

Shilts, Randy. *And the Band Played on: Politics, People, and the AIDS Epidemic*. New York: St. Martin's, 1987.

Sontag, Susan. *AIDS and Its Metaphors*. New York: Farrar, Straus and Giroux, 1988.

———. "The Way We Live Now." *The Houghton Mifflin Anthology of Short Fiction*. Edited by Patricia Hampl. Boston: Houghton Mifflin, 1989.

Whitmore, George. *Someone Was Here: Profiles in the AIDS Epidemic*. New York: New American Library, 1988.

Cholera

Duffy, John. *A History of Public Health in New York City, 1625–1866*. New York: Russell Sage Foundation, 1968.

Goodwin, Sarah Webster. "Poe's 'Masque of the Red Death' and the 'Dance of Death.'" In *Medievalism in American Culture: Special Studies*, 17–28. Edited by Bernard Rosenthal and Paul E. Szarmach. Binghamton: State University of New York, CEMERS, 1987.

Poe, Edgar Allan. *Selected Writings of Edgar Allan Poe*. Edited by Edward H. Davidson. Boston: Houghton Mifflin, 1956.

Reese, David M. *A Plain and Practical Treatise on the Epidemic Cholera As It Prevailed in the City of New York in the Summer of 1832*. New York, 1833.

Report of the Council of Hygiene and Public Health on the Citizens' Association of New York, Upon the Sanitary Condition of the City [1866]. New York: Arno, 1970.

Rosenberg, Charles E. *The Cholera Years: The United States in 1832, 1849, and 1866*. Chicago: University of Chicago Press, 1962.

Whitman, Walt. *Walt Whitman: The Early Poems and the Fiction*. Edited by Thomas L. Brasher. New York: New York University Press, 1963.

———. *Leaves of Grass*. Comprehensive Reader's Edition. Edited by Harold W. Blodgett and Scully Bradley. New York: W. W. Norton, 1965.

Influenza

Crosby, Alfred W. *America's Forgotten Pandemic: The Influenza of 1918*. Cambridge, Mass.: Harvard University Press, 1989.

Givner, Joan. *Katherine Anne Porter: A Life*. New York: Simon and Schuster, 1982.

Osborn, June E., ed. *Influenza in America, 1918–1976*. New York: Prodist, 1977.

Porter, Katherine Anne. *Pale Horse, Pale Rider: Three Short Novels*. New York: Harcourt, Brace, 1936.

Malaria

James, Henry. "Daisy Miller" [1879]. In *The Henry James Reader*. Edited by Leon Edel. New York: Scribner's, 1965.

Shryock. *Medicine and Society in America*. See under General.

Poliomyelitis

Paul, John Rodman. *A History of Poliomyelitis*. New Haven, Conn.: Yale University Press, 1971.
Smith, Jane S. *Patenting the Sun: Polio and the Salk Vaccine*. New York: Morrow, 1990.

Smallpox

Bercovitch, Sacvan. *The American Jeremiad*. Madison: University of Wisconsin Press, 1978.
Colacurcio, Michael J. *The Province of Piety: Moral History in Hawthorne's Early Tales*. Cambridge, Massachusetts: Harvard University Press, 1984.
Colman, Benjamin. *Some Observations on the New Method of Receiving the Smallpox by Engrafting or Inoculation, in New England*. Boston, 1721.
Douglass, William. *A Dissertation Concerning Inoculation of the Smallpox*. London, 1730.
———. *A Practical Essay Concerning the Smallpox*. Boston, 1730.
Duffy, John. *Epidemics in Colonial America*. Baton Rouge: Louisiana State University Press, 1953.
Fenner, F., et al. *Smallpox and Its Eradication*. Geneva: World Health Organization, 1988.
Hawthorne, Nathaniel. *Twice-Told Tales* [1837]. Columbus: Ohio State University Press, 1974.
Liebman, Sheldon W. "Ambiguity in 'Lady Eleanore's Mantle,' " *Emerson Society Quarterly* 58 (1970): 97–101.
Macaulay, Thomas Babington. *The History of England from the Accession of James II*, 4 vols. Philadelphia, 1887.
Miller, Perry. *The New England Mind: From Colony to Province*. Boston: Beacon, 1953.
Sappenfield, James A. *A Sweet Instruction: Franklin's Journalism as a Literary Apprenticeship*. Carbondale: Southern Illinois University Press, 1973.
Silverman, Kenneth. *The Life and Times of Cotton Mather*. New York: Columbia University Press, 1985.

Swine Flu

Silverstein, Arthur M. *Pure Politics and Impure Science: The Swine Flu Affair*. Baltimore: Johns Hopkins University Press, 1981.

Syphilis

Andreski, Stanislav. *Syphilis, Puritanism, and Witch Hunts*. New York: St. Martin's, 1989.
Jones, James H. *Bad Blood: The Tuskegee Syphilis Experiment*. New York: Free Press, 1981.

Tuberculosis

Alcott, Louisa May. *Little Women* [1868–69]. New York: World, 1969.
Beard, George. *A Practical Treatise on Nervous Exhaustion (neurasthenia). Its*

Symptoms, Nature, Sequences, Treatment [1905]. Edited by A. D. Rockwell. New York: Kraus Reprint, 1971.

Brown, E. Richard. *Rockefeller's Medicine Men: Medicine and Capitalism in America*. Berkeley: University of California Press, 1979.

Caldwell, Mark. *The Last Crusade: The War on Consumption, 1862–1954*. New York: Atheneum, 1988.

Cather, Willa. *Willa Cather's Collected Short Fiction, 1892–1912*. Edited by Virginia Faulkner. Lincoln: University of Nebraska Press, 1965.

Dietrickson, Jan W. *The Image of Money in the American Novel of the Gilded Age*. New York: Humanities Press, 1969.

Emerson, Ralph Waldo. *Selections from Ralph Waldo Emerson: An Organic Anthology*. Edited by Stephen E. Whicher. Boston: Houghton Mifflin, 1957.

———. *Journals and Miscellaneous Notebooks of Ralph Waldo Emerson*, 16 vols. Edited by William H. Gilman and J. E. Parsons. Vol. 8, 1841–1843. Cambridge, Mass.: Harvard University Press, 1970.

Fowler, Virginia C. *Henry James' American Girl: The Embroidery on the Canvas*. Madison: University of Wisconsin Press, 1984.

Gelb, Arthur and Barbara. *O'Neill*. New York: Harper & Row, 1962.

Harding, Walter. *The Days of Henry Thoreau: A Biography* [New York: Knopf, 1965]. New York: Dover, 1982.

James, Henry. *The Wings of the Dove*, New York Edition. New York: Scribner's, 1909.

———. *Henry James: Representative Selections*. Edited by Lyon N. Richardson. Urbana: University of Illinois Press, 1966.

———. *Henry James Letters*, 2 vols. Edited by Leon Edel. Vol. 1, 1843–1875. Cambridge, Mass.: Harvard University Press, 1974.

Lutz, Tom. *American Nervousness, 1903: An Anecdotal History*. Ithaca, N.Y.: Cornell University Press, 1991.

Mann, Thomas. *The Magic Mountain* [1924]. New York: Knopf, 1952.

Nowell, Elizabeth. *Thomas Wolfe: A Biography*. Garden City, N.Y.: Doubleday, 1960.

O'Neill, Eugene. *The Complete Plays* (Literary Classics of the United States). New York: Viking, 1988.

Parker, Theodore. *Life and Correspondence of Theodore Parker*, 2 vols. [1864]. Edited by John Weiss. Freeport, N.Y.: Books for Libraries Press, 1969.

Parsons, Talcott. "Health and Illness in the Light of American Values." *Concepts of Health and Disease: Interdisciplinary Perspectives*. Edited by Arthur L. Caplan, et al. Reading, Mass.: Addison-Wesley Publishing, 1981.

Rusk, Ralph L. *The Life of Ralph Waldo Emerson*. New York: Scribner's, 1949.

Stowe, Harriet Beecher. *Uncle Tom's Cabin, or, Life among the Lowly* [1852]. New York: Penguin American Library, 1981.

Strouse, Jean. *Alice James: A Biography*. Boston: Houghton Mifflin, 1980.

Thoreau, Henry David. *The Correspondence of Henry David Thoreau*. Edited by Walter Harding and Carl Bode. New York: New York University Press, 1958.

———. *The Writings of Henry David Thoreau* [1906], vol. 2. New York: AMS Press, 1968.

Wolfe, Thomas. *Look Homeward, Angel*. New York: Scribner's Modern Library, 1929.

Yellow Fever

Alexander, John K. "Poverty, Fear, and Continuity: An Analysis of the Poor in Late Eighteenth-Century Philadelphia." In *The Peoples of Philadelphia*, 13–35. Edited by Alan F. Davis and Mark H. Haller. Philadelphia: Temple University Press, 1973.

Bailey, Marcia E. *A Lesser Hartford Wit: Dr. Elihu Hubbard Smith*. Orono, Maine: The University Press, 1928.

Brown, Charles Brockden. *Arthur Mervyn, or, Memoirs of the Year 1793* [1799–1800]. Kent, Ohio: Kent State University Press, 1977.

———. *Ormond, or, The Secret Witness* [1799]. Kent, Ohio: Kent State University Press, 1982.

———. *Edgar Huntly, or, Memoirs of a Sleep-Walker* [1799]. Edited by Sydney J. Krause and S. W. Reid. Kent, Ohio: Kent State University Press, 1984.

Buffon, Comte de (George Louis Leclerc). *Histoire naturelle*, 44 vols. London, 1749–1804.

Cabel, George Washington. *The Creoles of Louisiana*. New York: Scribner's, 1884.

———. *The Grandissimes*. New York: Hill and Wang, 1957.

Cameron, Ian. *The Impossible Dream: The Building of the Panama Canal*. New York: Morrow, 1972.

Carey, Mathew. *A Short Account of the Malignant Fever Lately Prevalent in Philadelphia* . . . Philadelphia, 1793.

de Kruif, Paul. *Microbe Hunters*. New York: Blue Ribbon Books, 1926.

Delaport, Francois. *The History of Yellow Fever: An Essay on the Birth of Tropical Medicine*. Translated by Arthur Goldhammer. Cambridge, Mass.: MIT Press, 1991.

Dunlap, William. *The Life of Charles Brockden Brown*, 2 vols. Philadelphia, 1815.

Freneau, Philip. *The Poems of Philip Freneau*, vol. 3. Edited by Fred Lewis Pattee. Princeton, N.J.: Princeton University Library, 1907.

Howard, Sidney. *Yellow Jack*. New York: Harcourt, Brace, 1934.

Mack, Gerstle. *The Land Divided: A History of the Panama Canal*. New York: Octagon, 1974.

Marshall, William. *A Theological Dissertation on the Propriety of Removing from the Seat of the Pestilence*. Philadelphia, 1799.

Powell, John. *Bring Out Your Dead*. Philadelphia: University of Pennsylvania Press, 1949.

Rush, Benjamin. *An Account of the Bilious Remitting Yellow Fever As It Appeared in the City of Philadelphia in the Year 1793*. Philadelphia, 1794.

Smith, Elihu Hubbard. *A Collection of Papers on the Subject of Bilious Fevers Prevalent in the U.S. for a Few Years Past*. New York, 1796.

———. *The Diary of Elihu Hubbard Smith, 1771–1798*. Edited by James E. Cronin. Philadelphia: American Philosophical Society, 1973.

———. *The Medical Repository* 1 (February 1798).

Stevenson, Lloyd G. "Putting Disease on the Map: The Early Use of Spot Maps in the Study of Yellow Fever." *Journal of the History of Medicine and Allied Sciences* (vol. 20, 1965): 226–61.

Volney, C. F. *Tableau du climat et sol des Etats Unis* (A View of the Soil and

Climate of the United States of America). Translated by Charles Brockden
    Brown. New York: Hafner, 1968.
Webster, Noah. *A Brief History of Epidemical and Pestilential Diseases, with the
    Principal Phenomena of the Physical World Which Precede and Accompany
    Them* . . . [1799] (Burt Franklin Research and Source Works Series). New
    York: B. Franklin, 1970.
White, Sidney Howard. *Sidney Howard.* Boston: Twayne, 1977.
Wideman, John Edgar. *Fever: Twelve Stories.* New York: Henry Holt, 1989.

Index

ACT UP, 138, 139
Adams, Samuel Hopkins, 103
Adair, Peter: *Absolutely Positive*, 138
AIDS (acquired immune deficiency syndrome), 14, 15, 17, *125–47*, 148, 149; policies concerning, 130–32
Alcott, Louisa May, 90, 112; *Little Women*, 90–91
Alien and Sedition Acts, 53
Allen, Rt. Rev. Richard, 42, 45, 46, 56
American Medical Association (AMA), 101, 129

Barnett, Allen: *Body and Its Dangers, The*, 144; "The *Times* as It Knows Us," 144–45

Beard, George M., 118
Bentham, Jeremy, 3
Benton, Thomas Hart, 72–73
Billings, John Shaw, 101, 113
Boccaccio, Giovanni: *The Decameron*, 1
Boylston, Zabdiel, 27
Brackenridge, Hugh Henry, 50, 54
Brown, Charles Brockden, 4, 5, 42, 47, 49, 51–53, 60, 63, 64, 70, 80; *Arthur Mervyn*, 5, 48, 53, *57–59*, 64, 66, 67, 69, 141; *Edgar Huntly*, 5, 14, 48, 49, *64–69*; *Ormond*, 48, 49, 53, 57; *Wieland*, 48, 53, 58
Buffon, Comte de, 5, 6, 50; *Histoire naturelle*, 5

169

THE AUTHOR

Joann P. Krieg is associate professor of English at Hofstra University, Hempstead, New York. She teaches American literature and American studies and has published articles in both areas. Her edited volumes include *Walt Whitman: Here and Now* (1985) and *Robert Moses: Single-Minded Genius* (1989). She is also the author of a monograph, *Long Island and Literature* (1989), which reflects her interest in the connections between literature and landscape.